THE THERAPIST'S USE OF SELF

John Rowan
and
Michael Jacobs

Open University Press

Open University Press
McGraw-Hill Education
McGraw-Hill House
Shoppenhangers Road
Maidenhead
Berkshire
SL6 2QL

email: enquiries@openup.co.uk
world wide web: www.openup.co.uk

First Published 2002
Reprinted 2003, 2006, 2007, 2008

A catalogue record of this book is available from the British Library
ISBN-10 0 335 20776 6 (pb) 0 335 20777 4 (hb)
ISBN-13 978 0 335 20776 3 (pb) 978 0 335 20777 0 (hb)

Library of Congress Cataloging-in-Publication Data
Rowan, John.
    The therapist's use of self/John Rowan and Michael Jacobs.
      p. cm – (Core concepts in therapy)
    Includes bibliographical references and index.
    ISBN 0-335-20777-4 (hb) – ISBN 0-335-20776-6 (pbk.)
      1. Psychotherapy. 2. Psychotherapist and patient.
      3. Psychotherapists–Psychology. I. Jacobs, Michael, 1941- II. Title.
    III. Series.
  RC480.5 .R69 2002
  616.89'14–dc21

                                                        2002023852

Typeset by Graphicraft Limited, Hong Kong
Printed in Great Britain by Bell & Bain Ltd., Glasgow

THE THERAPIST'S USE OF SELF

Core concepts in therapy

Series editor: Michael Jacobs

Over the last ten years a significant shift has taken place in the relations between representatives of different schools of therapy. Instead of the competitive and often hostile reactions we once expected from each other, therapists from different points of the spectrum of approaches are much more interested in where they overlap and where they differ. There is a new sense of openness to cross-orientation learning.

The Core Concepts in Therapy series compares and contrasts the use of similar terms across a range of the therapeutic models, and seeks to identify where different terms appear to denote similar concepts. Each book is authored by two therapists, each one from a distinctly different orientation; and, where possible, each one from a different continent, so that an international dimension becomes a feature of this network of ideas.

Each of these short volumes examines a key concept in psychological therapy, setting out comparative positions in a spirit of free and critical enquiry, but without the need to prove one model superior to another. The books are fully referenced and point beyond themselves to the wider literature on each topic.

Forthcoming and published titles:

Contents

Series editor's preface

A major aspect of intellectual and cultural life in the twentieth century has been the study of psychology – present, of course, for many centuries in practical form and expression in the wisdom and insight to be found in spirituality, in literature and in the dramatic arts, as well as in arts of healing and guidance, both in the East and West. In parallel with the deepening interest in the inner processes of character and relationships in the novel and theatre in the nineteenth century, psychiatry reformulated its understanding of the human mind, and encouraged, in those brave enough to challenge the myths of mental illness, new methods of exploration of psychological processes.

The second half of the twentieth century witnessed an explosion of interest both in theories about personality, psychological development, cognition and behaviour, and in the practice of therapy, or perhaps more accurately, the therapies. It also saw, as is common in any intellectual discipline, battles between theories and therapists of different persuasions, particularly between psychoanalysis and behavioural psychology, and each in turn with humanistic and transpersonal therapies, as well as within the major schools themselves. If such arguments are not surprising, and indeed objectively can be seen as healthy – potentially promoting greater precision in research, alternative approaches to apparently intractable problems, and deeper understanding of the wellsprings of human thought, emotion and behaviour – it is nonetheless disturbing that, for many decades, there was so much sniping and entrenchment of positions from therapists who should have been able to look more closely at their own responses and rivalries. It is as if diplomats had ignored their skills and knowledge and resorted in their dealings with each other to gun slinging.

The psychotherapeutic enterprise has also been an international one. There were many centres of innovation, even at the beginning – Paris, Moscow, Vienna, Berlin, Zurich, London, Boston USA – and soon Edinburgh, Rome, New York, Chicago and California saw the development of different theories and therapeutic practice. Geographical location has added to the richness of the discipline, in particular identifying cultural and social differences, and widening the psychological debate to include, at least in some instances, sociological and political dimensions.

The question has to be asked, given the separate developments due to location, research interests, personal differences and splits between and within traditions, whether what has sometimes been called 'psycho-babble' is indeed a welter of different languages describing the same phenomena through the particular jargon and theorizing of the various psychotherapeutic schools? Or are there genuine differences, which may lead sometimes to the conclusion that one school has got it right, while another has therefore got it wrong; or that there are 'horses for courses'; or, according to the Dodo principle, that 'all shall have prizes'?

The latter part of the twentieth century saw some rapprochement between the different approaches to the theory and practice of psychotherapy (and counselling), often due to the external pressures towards organizing the profession responsibly and to the high standards demanded of it by health care, by the public and by the state. It is out of this budding rapprochement that there came the motivation for this series, in which a number of key concepts that lie at the heart of the psychotherapies can be compared and contrasted across the board. Some of the terms used in different traditions may prove to represent identical concepts; others may look similar, but in fact highlight quite different emphases, which may or may not prove useful to those who practise from a different perspective. Other terms, apparently identical, may prove to mean something completely different in two or more schools of psychotherapy.

To carry out this project, it seemed essential that as many of the psychotherapeutic traditions as possible should be represented in the authorship of the series. To promote both this and the spirit of dialogue between the traditions, it also appeared desirable that there should be two authors for each book, each one representing, where practicable, different orientations. It was important that the series should be truly international in its approach and, therefore, in its authorship. And that miracle of late twentieth-century technology, the Internet, proved to be a productive means of finding authors, as well as a remarkably efficient method of communicating, in the cases of some pairs of authors, half-way across the world.

This series therefore represents, in a new millennium, an extremely exciting development, one which as series editor I have found more and more enthralling as I have eavesdropped on the drafts shuttling back and forth between authors. Here, for the first time, the reader will find all the major concepts of all the principal schools of psychotherapy and counselling (and not a few minor ones) drawn together so that they may be compared, contrasted and (it is my hope) above all used – used for the ongoing debate between orientations, but more importantly still, used for the benefit of clients and patients who are not at all interested in partisan positions, but in what works, or in what throws light upon their search for healing and understanding.

Michael Jacobs

Preface

Like most of the other pairings of authors in this series, we come from different theoretical orientations. It was never a foregone conclusion that we would see eye to eye, but as we acknowledge in the final chapter, we have in fact learned much from each other in the writing of this book. And we can take some pleasure from our awareness that we have respected each other's different emphases, which inevitably colour the way we have interpreted material from our own and other orientations. In the first five chapters, we have presented as objective an argument as it is possible to do, given the normal bias in any writer. But we have had each other to prevent excesses of enthusiasm for a particular approach! Although our individual intellectual and practical preferences no doubt slip in from time to time, we have tried to reserve our own views for the dialogue in Chapter 6, where something of the discussion that has taken place between us in the course of writing becomes more obvious to the reader.

What we did not know, despite our researches, we could not obviously share with each other or with the reader. Bertrand Russell is said to have replied to a question, what he would tell God if after death he found himself before the judgement seat, 'Why didn't you make it clearer?' We make no claims to omniscience, and it is certain that we have not covered everything that has been written on the subject. And while we own all shortcomings in this book as our own, if there are significant omissions it may also be because some orientations have not made as clear as *we* would have wished where they stand on the therapist's use of self.

We have each valued working with another person who takes meticulous care in getting the wording right, who ensures even in the draft stage that references (so important in a book such as this) are up-to-date and accurate, and who promptly returns amended material to the other. It has felt like a good model of cooperative work. The many references to the literature on the subject demonstrate how much we owe to those who have written on the topic. It has not been our primary aim to be original, but rather to record as accurately as possible the thinking about this set of concepts related to the use of the self in therapy. Nevertheless, we hope that the particular approach we have taken gives the subject some originality in its presentation.

John Rowan
Michael Jacobs

CHAPTER 1

Introduction

My therapist is chaotic – well, in one sense chaotic. Sessions seldom start on time because he always runs over with the previous client; but then he runs over with me, too, so I forgive him for that. His consulting room is a mess – papers all over the floor and falling off the desk. And when we start, as I often do, with some mindless chatter, he joins in for a while. But then he stops and listens, and I sink into the chair and it all spills out. He is just the most marvellous listener. When he speaks it's again a bit of a muddle, and I'm not sure what he's really saying. But somehow what matters most is that he's listened to me.

My therapist is very precise. We start and finish right on time, and I value that, because I know when I have to start getting ready to put on my 'outside world' face. She sits quietly behind the couch, but I know she's there, because her presence is strong. I don't want her to say much, but I do want her to be there. I know nothing about her, but that doesn't matter, because the time is for me and that's something I really need. There's so much pain in me, that for the moment I know that what I want is someone to accept it, hold it, but not try and smooth it over with kind words or clever explanations.

I didn't think counsellors said much, but mine says quite a lot, although when I come to think about it what she says is nearly always what she thinks I am saying, or what she feels about what's going on in the ether, as it were, between me and her and her and me. She sometimes tells me about herself, but only when it ties in with something I've said, or tried to say, about me; and it helps enormously to know that she understands from her own experience just what I'm going through. And if she goes on, as she sometimes does, what I really like is that I can tell her she's taking over my time. And that's really important, that there's give and take in the session, and we can be really honest with each other.

What are therapists like? How do they work? Who are they behind the role? How far are therapists really like the way they are told to be in books? It is tempting to think of them as being very similar, clones of, for example, Freud, Rogers or Ellis, adhering to set patterns of understanding, relating, responding and reacting. But as anyone who has seen more than one therapist or counsellor can tell you, they are very different (except those who are indeed clones and who seem only to be acting a part, doing what they were told to do in their training). It is not just that therapists of various orientations work differently, since that is what we might expect. It is that within the same orientation each practitioner has developed (except for the clones, who have *put on*) a particular style, a way of being, a way of expressing themselves that is congruent with their approach, with the individual patient or client, and with his or her own self.

We record above three quite different experiences of therapists, all of which, for those patients, appear to work: they 'fit' without appearing to have become collusive. Traditionally, the Freudian therapist has hidden behind the couch and been quite unknown to the client; the person-centred therapist has been consistently positive, speaking in warm tones, deeply empathizing with the client, repeating words and phrases with extra meaning; and the behavioural psychologist has a clipboard with a checklist of questions and carefully worked out instructions for exercises to be practised now and outside the session. But is that really tradition, or is it myth, based on caricatures and stereotypes often thrown up by those who only imagine what such therapists are like?

Although it was not always recognized as such in the beginning, and for a while became submerged beneath all the debates about technique and psychopathology, it has become clear that the key to the talking therapies – and, indeed, perhaps to other forms of therapy – is the therapeutic relationship (Clarkson 1995). It is a necessary part of the therapy, although not always sufficient. Different orientations have discussed the therapeutic relationship using a large compendium of terms, sometimes similarly – empathy comes to mind – and sometimes in distinct ways that appear to have little in common. A good deal of the thinking about the therapeutic relationship in psychoanalysis has come under the headings of 'countertransference' and 'projective identification'; much of the thinking in the humanistic approaches has come under such headings as 'self-disclosure', 'empathy', 'genuineness', 'non-possessive warmth', 'presence', 'personhood' and the like. These two streams of thinking have had the most to contribute to thinking about the therapist's own self, and they provide much material for this book, although we shall see how cognitive-behavioural therapy, transpersonal therapy, group and family therapy each has a position on the use of self that finds a place in one or more of the chapters. Nor must we forget the Jungian view that the therapist is just as much 'in' the process as is the patient (Jung 1966: 72–4). Other aspects of the therapist also enter the picture, including the way a therapist is trained and uses supervision to make greater use of her or his own reactions and responses and experience in working with any one patient or client.

This book concentrates on the part the therapist plays in the therapeutic relationship, not by way of techniques (see the companion volume on *Interventions and Techniques*: Seiser and Wastell 2002), or in the creation of a therapeutic environment (Hazler and Barwick 2001), or by way of theories of personality development (Simanowitz and Pearce, forthcoming), but by the use of the self: whether covertly (through self-monitoring and the deployment of inner attitudes and aptitudes) or more openly (through disclosure). The concept of the self is a complex one, but the arguments around this concept are the subject of another volume in the series (Brinich and Shelley 2002). This book will not explore the different ways in which the 'self' can be understood, although distinctions between true and false self in the therapist, and our descriptions of the instrumental, authentic and transpersonal self of the therapist, are nevertheless important ones. Our emphasis will be on the descriptors rather than what the self specifically may mean.

Three ways of being a therapist

The series of which this volume is part aims to consider core concepts across a wide variety of theoretical and practice orientations. Many of the companion volumes elect to do this by dividing up the chapters along theoretical lines: psychodynamic, humanistic, cognitive-behavioural, and so on. In our own discussions, we thought that such a plan would not do justice to the commonalities and the differences not only between but also within the different schools. It is not so much that there are *alternative* ways of being a therapist, of using the self. There are, rather, different ways in which most therapists might be able to use the self, which are not mutually exclusive. Arising out of the debate over whether psychotherapy is an art (or perhaps a craft) or a science, there is the equally interesting question as to what kind of expert the therapist is. In this book, we say that there are three main possibilities for this: the therapist's position can be instrumental, authentic or transpersonal. Each of these possibilities makes different assumptions about the self, about the relationship and about the level of consciousness involved in doing therapy. This, in turn, leads to different assumptions about the content of training and the process of supervision.

Note that we call these 'possibilities' or 'positions': they may often be referred to as 'levels', but we do not wish to suggest that any one is superior to another. The reason why many people are suspicious of the idea of levels or stages is that they think this means a hierarchy, and they are – as good democratic thinkers – suspicious of the whole idea of hierarchies. But it is perhaps worthwhile to make a distinction between domination hierarchies and actualization hierarchies, as Eisler (1987) does. The term 'domination hierarchies', she says, is used to describe hierarchies based on force or the express or implied threat of force, which are characteristic of the human rank orderings in male-dominated societies. But such hierarchies, she says, are very different from the types of hierarchies found in progressions from lower to higher orderings of functioning, such as the progression from cells to organs in living organisms, for example. These latter types of hierarchies, which represent an evolutionary process, she urges, may be characterized by the term 'actualization hierarchies' because their function is to maximize the organism's potentials. By contrast, as evidenced by both sociological and psychological studies, human hierarchies based on force or the threat of force not only inhibit personal creativity, but also result in social systems in which the lowest (basest) human qualities are reinforced and humanity's higher aspirations (traits such as compassion and empathy as well as the striving for truth and justice) are systematically suppressed. The implication of all this is that domination hierarchies are indeed to be feared, but actualization hierarchies are benign. Each time we use concepts like levels or stages we have to look closely at what is being said, and which type of hierarchy is being invoked.

While recognizing that there can be good and bad practice in any of these levels or positions, we suggest that these possibilities will come into being through a subtle combination of the confidence and development of the therapist, and the needs of the client and the place where the client currently is. These three separate positions form the subject of each of the next three chapters, and are examined again in Chapter 5, where we look at the relevance of these possibilities for training and supervision. In the final chapter, we move away from our best efforts to present the model objectively, and discuss our own views on the implications of our study on being a therapist. To present our model as an overview before going into detail, we summarize the three positions here.

In the *instrumental* position, the client is usually regarded as someone who has problems, which need to be put right (by the client, by the therapist or by both); this can lead to the therapist acting in a somewhat programmed way. Technical ability is regarded as something both possible and desirable. In rational emotive behaviour therapy, in neuro-linguistic programming and in many cognitive-behavioural approaches, this is the preferred mode; and the treatment approaches in vogue under managed care and employee assistance programmes often take a similar view. Specific techniques have to be learned and put into practice in time-limited work, for example, which nearly always include identification of a clear focus or problem. The client or patient is there to be cured, at least in this one identifiable respect, and application of the correct techniques aims to achieve this in a high percentage of cases. More and better techniques are the way forward, and to test these objectively is the main goal of research. Working with the unconscious can be just as much part of this approach as not working with the unconscious. It is equally possible here for the relationship to be long or short, close or distant, self-disclosing or anonymous, using transference or not, involving bodywork or not, political or not, analytic or humanistic, cognitive or emotive, or otherwise. The key thing is that there should be an aim. Every form of therapy resorts to this level of working at times, and the famed Working Alliance is firmly based on it, but it is basically an I–It relationship rather than an I–Thou relationship, in the terms made famous by Martin Buber (1970). Key words here are 'contract', 'assessment', 'treatment goals', 'empirically validated treatments', 'boundaries' and 'manualization'. In Chapter 2, we concentrate on this approach and this form of therapist identity.

In the *authentic* way of being, personal involvement is much more acceptable, with the therapist much more closely identified with the client and more openly concerned to explore the therapeutic relationship. The idea of the wounded healer is often mentioned, as is the idea of personal growth. The schools who most traditionally and obviously favour this approach are the humanistic ones: person-centred, gestalt, psychodrama, bodywork, focusing, experiential, existential, and so on. Yet there is also considerable evidence that, under different names, this same type of relationship is very important to many psychoanalytic therapists and even more, perhaps, to Jungians and post-Jungians. Clarkson (1995) calls it the person-to-person relationship. Again it is possible to work in this way whether one believes in the unconscious or not. According to one's theoretical position, to work in this way it is essential to have had some experience of what Wilber (2000) calls the Centaur level of psychospiritual development, or what Wade (1996) calls authentic consciousness. Again the analytic model may express it quite differently, but concepts of countertransference in more recent usage are significant here and depend upon the openness of the therapist to such intuitive information. Key words here are 'authenticity', 'personhood', 'healing through meeting', 'being in the world', 'intimacy', 'openness' and 'the real relationship'. We discuss the authentic way of being and working in Chapter 3.

In the *transpersonal* way of being, the boundaries between therapist and client may fall away. Both may occupy the same space at the same time, at the level of what is sometimes termed 'soul', sometimes 'heart' and sometimes 'essence': what they have in common is a willingness to let go of all aims and all assumptions. Clarkson (1995) is clear that this is one of the five important relationships that have to be acknowledged in therapy. What she does not make clear, however, is that to adopt this way of working it is essential to have had some experience of what Wilber (2000) calls the 'Subtle' level of psychospiritual development, or what Buddhists call the *Sambhogakaya*. Again here it is necessary to look for parallels outside the discourse of transpersonal or spiritual therapies, and these we shall observe, as in the analyst Bion's (1965) 'O'. Key words here are 'interbeing', 'linking', 'transcendental empathy', 'resonance', 'dual unity', 'communion', 'the four-dimensional state' and 'ultimate reality'. In Chapter 4, we examine these approaches in more detail. It is the least well known of the three positions we have identified.

Each of these positions is based on a good deal of evidence. Since in the chapters that follow we concentrate more on the content of each position rather than justifying the position itself, we can briefly outline here the background thinking to our choice of this approach.

The *instrumental* is described by Maslow (1987) as the motivational position where people need the esteem of others. It is described by Kohlberg (1981) and his co-worker Gilligan (1982) as the conventional moral level and by Loevinger (1976) in her work on women and girls as the conformist level of ego development. Wade (1996) sees it as the (mainly masculine) achievement level and as the (mainly feminine) affiliative level of personal development. Belenky and her co-workers (1986) call it the level of procedural knowing; Wilber (2000) describes it as the Mental Ego level of psychospiritual development. All these investigators are, of course, using a stage model of development, as do other well-known names, such as Piaget (1950) and Erikson (1965). Such well-researched models have been found to be very useful in education, management training and social science generally.

The *authentic* is described by these same authors as self-actualization (Maslow), post-conventional moral positions (Kohlberg), true personal conscience (Gilligan), autonomous and integrated ego development (Loevinger), authentic consciousness (Wade), constructed knowing (Belenky) and the Centaur stage (Wilber). So again there is a mass of research supporting the importance of such a level of development. There is also a rich variety of philosophical thinking that illuminates our knowledge of this level. Heidegger (1962) makes the distinction between authentic and inauthentic, which has been so influential here. Sartre (1948) has been even more pointed in his insistence that authenticity is very special and has to be taken seriously in its existential implications. The person who has done most, perhaps, to naturalize the notion of authenticity into the realm of therapy is Bugental (1981), although Binswanger (1963) and May (1980) also made important contributions. This way of being is within the range of experience open to all of us. We shall see in Chapter 3 that it is strongly prevalent among the theorists within the field of therapy.

The *transpersonal* is less familiar than the other two possibilities and many of the writers mentioned do not go this far; but an increasing number of therapists find it necessary, as we shall see in Chapter 4. From the vantage point of what Wilber calls the Subtle, it becomes clear that the authentic way is limited by having strict boundaries. At the Subtle level, talk about boundaries becomes much more problematic. Wilber's (1981) own book on therapy is entitled *No Boundary*, and this is clearly quite central to the thinking at this stage. Stanislav Grof has written a series of important books in this field (e.g. Grof 1988), and two books that link therapy with the transpersonal are Cortright (1997) and West (2000). A number of post-Jungians have made important contributions to the area, such as Hillman (1996) and Schwartz-Salant (1984, 1991). Boorstein (1996) has edited a book of readings on transpersonal psychotherapy. *The Journal of Transpersonal Psychology, The International Journal of Transpersonal Studies* and, in Britain, *The Transpersonal Psychology Review*, published by the British Psychological Society, are useful sources. One of the best books in this area is the one on transcultural counselling and spirituality by Fukuyama and Sevig (1999), which spells out in some detail how spirituality integrates with therapy when working with clients from other cultures. Other interesting books in this area are Brazier's (2001) *Zen Therapy* and Epstein's (1996) *Thoughts Without a Thinker*. The title of the latter, a phrase of Bion's (1992: 326), shows another example of where psychoanalysis too, once thought to be formalized and rigid in its thinking and practice, also has a voice or two reflecting on this position.

Indeed, it has been our experience in researching and writing that we have found significant parallels running through the three possible ways of being that we describe. That has been enriching for us both as authors and therapists, and leads us to hope that our text may also enhance the therapist's use of self for our various readers.

C H A P T E R 2

The instrumental self

As stated in the Introduction, this chapter deals with therapy as a set of skills that can be learned and applied. Some may feel that this is more the case in counselling than in psychotherapy, but with the range of therapies now available, this approach is just as common in the field of psychotherapy. There are now many, both in, for example, the British National Health Service and outside it, who are being taught this approach and who are practising it every day. The therapist is taught how to adopt a therapist persona, or a therapist role, and to practise it skilfully and effectively.

As an example, a therapist might choose to use questionnaires as part of the therapy. Indeed, it is interesting that, in the parallel series to *Core Concepts in Therapy*, several of the contributors, from quite different orientations, use such questionnaires at an early stage (Dryden 1995; Lapworth 1995; Margison 1995; Millar 1995; Ormrod 1995; Ryle 1995). Such an approach definitely falls into the category of the instrumental, where the questionnaire is an instrument, which on its own would be impersonal and, so to speak, 'no respecter of persons'.

Furthermore, the issues that we identify in this chapter bear on the debate about whether psychotherapy is an art (or perhaps a craft) or a science, which, in turn, has some bearing on the discussion between cognitive-behavioural therapies and psychoanalytic and humanistic therapies as to the purpose of therapy – is it to mend the mind in the machine, or is it to promote deeper understanding and/or growth of something much more vaguely called 'the person'? In addition, we are aware that what we are dealing with here involves the debate between classical psychoanalytic technique and much humanistic understanding of the role of the therapist – what kind of expert is the therapist? An expert in fathoming the deeper reaches of the unconscious, where there may be an argument for an objectivity that also encourages regression, or an expert in relating in the here-and now, so encouraging progression?

Learning and applying the skills of therapy

Although both psychoanalysis and behaviour therapy at one stage might have fought over the most effective technique, they might have agreed that it was what the therapist does, rather than as a person-centred therapist would argue, who the therapist is, that matters. Yet even if research appears to find less significance in technique, and more in the quality of the relationship in psychotherapy and counselling (Clarkson 1995), there is still the question of whether what the therapist does is to engage in a certain role – one which is 'put on' for the therapy session – or whether the therapist should be totally engaged in the interaction, from within her or his inner self, rather than adopting a persona. Here we are concerned principally with those approaches, or aspects of otherwise different approaches, which hold the assumption that a role is involved in being a therapist, and that it is this that has to be learned.

It is not our brief to examine the techniques used in different therapies, that is the subject of the companion volume in this series on *Interventions and Techniques* (Seiser and Wastell 2002). But we are interested in whether the therapist uses herself or himself as one aspect of technique, as something instrumental. Such a view suggests that a therapist trains the self to become a therapeutic instrument, which is turned on and off at will. If this appears cynical, we can perhaps put it more positively by asking how a therapist might act if, driving to the consulting room, he or she has been involved in a series of mishaps and incidents, resulting in the therapist opening the waiting room door in a foul mood. He or she probably reveals none of this to the client, but instead greets the client as normal, and puts to one side the earlier events of the day for the duration of the session. Once the client has left the room, the therapist may pick up the phone and sound off to the car insurers, a partner, or some other person who lends an ear. But at the start of the second session, the mask is once more slipped over her or his feelings, and the session proceeds with the client none the wiser as to the emotional turmoil in the therapist.

This is not hard to imagine. It is not a deceitful act to put on the mask of the calm therapist. But it is nonetheless a persona, a mask in the sense used by Jung (1968; Samuels 1985: 30–2) – that is, the actor's mask in classical theatre. It is a way of being the therapist has probably learned to adopt in training, as well as through experience of what is in the best interests of clients. Self-control is essential when personal feelings run high, and training aims at enabling therapists to be more 'in charge' of their own emotions. Training also gives the therapist a basic way of talking that is likely to pertain to the theory being taught and to the actual school where the training takes place.

Nevertheless, we might also ask how the therapist would respond were the client, in our imagined scenario, to observe that the therapist looks fraught. Lomas, for example, writing from a perspective critical of psychoanalytic technique, though himself psychodynamic in his position, might well respond on a personal level (see, in a similar situation, Lomas 1981: 67–8); a person-centred therapist would probably respond similarly, placing a premium on congruence (Mearns and Thorne 1988: 76–81); and an existentialist therapist likewise, stressing authenticity.

In addition, therapy usually involves the use of definite skills, and the training of therapists might involve the inculcation of micro-skills, as Ivey *et al.* (1987) have urged. The emphasis here in the learning of the trainee therapist is clearly on certain technical aspects, rather than on the personal alone; and changes in learned behaviour and in usual social skills may well be necessary. In one sense, therapists may not quite be able to be 'themselves' in the way they would be used to in, for example, debating an issue with an intellectual adversary or engaging in a conversation on a street corner. But the self that the trainee therapist is invited to develop is nevertheless a type of act, a form of role-playing: to listen rather than interrupt as they otherwise might in an argument; to accept without passing judgement, where in another situation they might want to challenge a moral position; to select a response carefully, rather than spontaneously react. We are not suggesting that learning to play a different role is wrong, or even false. It is possible that making such cognitive and behavioural changes in the way they react will have a deeper effect on trainee therapists, and make them more sensitive, less judgemental and better listeners in relationships generally, as Kennedy and Charles (1989: 62) have argued: 'Maturing counsellors appreciate the fact that what they do in counselling does not ask them to change themselves as much as it invites them to come closer to their best and frequently unrealised selves'. But equally it might be argued that there is nothing wrong with being quite different in the consulting room from the way one is outside it. It might even be in order, particularly for those who see therapy as being about a learned technique, to tell lies to the client, or (to put a more positive gloss on it) to be 'economical with the truth' if it were felt to be therapeutic and in the present interests of the client. Although Mearns and Thorne (1988: 84) cite examples of hiding negative feelings about the client as incongruent, Winnicott (1975: 196) provides a good example of holding back his negative feelings until his patient was ready to hear them.

In systemic therapy with families, there has been a move towards recognizing that we cannot understand the view of an observer or therapist without taking into account their own position within the system. This means recognizing the ways in which the beliefs and experience of the therapist influence the process of therapy. This shift in emphasis, away from the view of the therapist as an impartial observer, has some connection with the concepts of transference and countertransference, but differs in that it does not necessarily postulate that this operates at an unconscious level. The effect of this is that most systemic therapists include greater emphasis on their use of self in sessions than previously. However, the position taken up is very much that of the expert who can see the situation more clearly than those involved directly.

We do not suggest an absolute dichotomy between the therapist's use of self as a kind of persona, which forms the basis for this chapter, and the therapist's attempt to use the true self, which is the basis for the next. Both may apply. For example, we may appear to suggest that the person-centred approach would support only the genuine use of the inner self of the therapist and would eschew the 'persona' self that we describe here. However, take this short extract from one of Carl Rogers' most important articles:

> The fifth condition is that the therapist is experiencing an accur-
> ate, empathic understanding of the client's awareness of his
> own experience. To sense the client's private world as if it were
> your own, but without ever losing the 'as if' quality – that is
> empathy, and this seems essential to therapy. To sense the
> client's anger, fear, or confusion as if it were your own, yet
> without your own anger, fear or confusion getting bound up in
> it, is the condition we are endeavouring to describe.
>
> (Rogers 1957: 99)

Here Rogers describes a conscious and deliberate act on the part of the therapist, to put himself or herself into the client's private world, but at the same time not allow personal feelings to get caught up in the client's experience. The 'as if' quality puts it well, but of course suggests that being empathic, however genuine in its endeavours, does mean putting part of the therapist's true self and own experience to one side. We return to this type of empathy in the third section of this chapter. The 'as if' reminds us again of the actor's role in theatre and the mask or persona. Perhaps in Rogers' intention this would best be described as a position somewhere between the persona and the true self. Generally, it is quite hard to find in the humanistic and existential tradition examples of the view that the therapist is mainly an instrument, although Gerard Egan (1994) perhaps comes closest to it.

Elsewhere, Mearns and Thorne (2000) raise the issue from the person-centred tradition of the trend in the counselling and psychotherapy profession towards proving its effectiveness to attract public and medical insurance funding, both in the United States and in Britain, which results in what these authors call the manualization of treatment, as if the delivery of therapy is the same as using a car maintenance manual. Henry *et al.* (1993) found in their research that therapists in training who adhered to a manualized psychodynamic model adversely affected the therapeutic relationship, leading to an increase of hostility by the therapists towards clients.

Closely allied to this is the popular idea that there is a correct way of responding, seen in the many publications about counselling skills, although of course such books identify different responses rather than suggest exactly what might be said (Jacobs 2000b). There might even, given some series of books on different presenting problems, appear to be a 'best way' of tackling each issue brought to therapy. It is an interesting question whether this promotes the importance of research to test these ideas or whether it is research that promotes such an attitude; but it is easy to see, when research findings appear to demonstrate that, for example, certain techniques prove most effective with phobias, how therapists are then encouraged to learn and to use such techniques and to promote them with their clients. Research can then be used to guide therapy and may encourage the idea that the therapist should follow a manual of tried and tested skills.

The pressure to prove efficacy leads to the need to define what steps in therapy are taken and when, which, in turn, is reflected in Britain in the acceptance by counselling of competency driven training, as if (in the eyes of the scheme for National Vocational Qualifications and their Scottish equivalent) counselling were the same as learning any other trade. The concern shown in person-centred practitioners about reducing counselling to 'surface relational competencies such as clarifying, not interrupting, listening, summarising and asking open-ended questions' (Mearns and Thorne 2000: 40) has been reflected in the psychoanalytic tradition in Britain, also highly suspicious of attempts to define therapy in terms of competencies. Training manuals that identify what we have already referred to above as micro-skills run the risk of inculcating similar attitudes in tutors and students, who in assessing competency generally may concentrate upon those readily identifiable skills. These are easier to quantify than what can be called 'higher-level skills' such as 'meeting the client at relational depth' (Mearns 1996, 1997), a phrase that would be echoed in many other orientations than just the person-centred. However, we take it for granted that the teaching and learning of skills is legitimate and useful, as described for example in an excellent chapter by Inskipp (2000).

If research into psychotherapy was at one time almost confined to behavioural (and later to cognitive-behavioural) forms of therapy, this approach is also now to be found among the psychoanalysts and the humanistic practitioners. Langs (1982), for example, in the psychoanalytic tradition, interprets the unconscious communication of the patient in such a detailed way as to promote an acutely conscious mental attitude in the therapist, constantly translating the patient's communications in an endeavour to understand what is really being said. Here a place for the therapist's own responses could easily get lost, and the unconscious reduced to something that can be studied mathematically. Lake (1966), in the humanistic and transpersonal tradition, wanted to make much more precise the path by which diagnostic categories emerged, and his charts are a model of reducing complex realities to something more intellectually manageable.

As might be expected in the cognitive-behavioural approach, the pendulum swings more obviously towards the therapist playing a role. Such an approach appears to view the therapist in a purely functional way, more as an educator than as someone who engages at a feeling level in the process. Take rational emotive behaviour therapy (REBT), for example:

REBT therapists see themselves as good psychological educators and therefore seek to teach their clients the ABC model of

understanding and dealing with their psychological problems . . .
REBT therapists frequently employ an active-directive counselling
style and use both Socratic and didactic teaching methods.

(Dryden 2000: 329)

There is a theoretical basis for this, in that no distinction is made
between the ego and the self, and the self is therefore treated just
like an ego. Since the ego is role-bounded and is in need of discipline and order, there is nothing wrong with treating it like an
instrument. Ellis, for example, is very clear about this (Ellis and
Yeager 1989).

Newer traditions, such as neuro-linguistic programming (NLP),
follow the same trend:

The skills needed by the NLP practitioner can be thought of from
three perspectives – conceptual, analytical and behavioural. Conceptual skills include the understanding of, and ability to apply,
NLP conceptual models. Analytical skills include the ability to
analyse the system (including the practitioner's own and the
client's behaviour) in terms of its component parts. Behavioural
skills include the practitioner's ability to vary their own behaviour to influence the system and to facilitate the client's ability
to change.

(Cooper and Seal 2000: 391)

The therapist is supposed to be infinitely malleable, able to turn the
self (or ego) into any form required ('there are no impossible clients
– only inefficient therapists'). There is or should be no resistance to
this.

Similarly, in the systemic tradition, no distinction is made between
the self of the therapist and the role being played. Like the patients,
the therapist and the team are seen as simply parts of a larger whole.
Sometimes, indeed, the therapist becomes just an instrument of the
team, following orders given by them.

In the psychodynamic tradition, things are more complex. Some
theorists, including Rangell (1954), Waelder (1960), Kernberg (1975),
Brenner (1976) and Gaskill (1980), have treated the unconscious of
the therapist as a tool, something to be ordered and disciplined. For
such theorists, the main purpose of the training analysis is to reduce
the self of the therapist, both conscious and unconscious, to something usable technically. Only when this is done can the analyst
deal adequately with the unconscious mechanisms involved:

Psychoanalysis is a method of therapy *whereby* conditions are brought about favorable for the development of a transference neurosis, in which the past is restored in the present, *in order that*, through a systematic interpretative attack on the resistances which oppose it, there occurs a resolution of that neurosis (trans-ference *and* infantile) *to the end* of bringing about structural changes in the mental apparatus of the patient to make the latter capable of optimum adaptation to life.
                              (Rangell 1954: 739–40, emphasis added)

One must never be at the mercy of one's unconscious mind. Psy-choanalytic approaches have certainly been characterized as more concerned with theoretical models and technique, even if there has been recognition of the blocking effect of therapists who have not been able to work through their personal material sufficiently to be open to the patient's communications. It is this concern that ini-tially identified what is known as countertransference, and led to the training analysis as a way of diminishing its influence in the conduct of therapy. Other aspects of psychoanalytic training have sometimes resulted in unquestioning obedience to certain techniques and, indeed, to a lack of training in the micro-skills of relating.

All the views of the therapist's use of self expressed in this chapter fit with what, in the transpersonal tradition, Wilber (1980a) calls the Mental Ego. Here the phrase is taken quite literally. The self or ego of the therapist is something to be used. The whole attitude is in-strumental, because the work of the therapist is essentially seen as a role. Everything can be understood, everything can be described, everything can be taught and everything can be learned. This is a confident and enterprising approach to the world, which democratic-ally opens everything up for intelligent examination. The basic mental model is of a controlling intellect moulding and training a possibly recalcitrant set of emotions, bodily reactions, unconscious responses or whatever else.

Therefore, in each of the major orientations, we find those who take the view that the therapist needs to be trained to be technically sound, to have a well-ordered mind that is not clouded by personal material; to be able to use research to develop techniques that will prove more efficacious in achieving the particular goals of the therapy; and to use supervision with the objective of becoming more accur-ate in understanding of the client's material and more precise in responding to it. Such a view has implications not just for the relationship between the therapist and the client, but also for the attention paid to the therapist's internal processes and the development of these in training and supervision (see Chapter 5).

While we examine training and supervision in Chapter 5, the element of training known as personal therapy arose in the psychoanalytic tradition partly from concern to free the analyst from the effects of countertransference. We perhaps put it crudely to suggest that the requirement for personal analysis lent support to the notion of the therapist as technician, but in the next section of this chapter we use the initial understanding of countertransference to begin to draw a distinction between the therapist as someone set apart from the client, and the therapist (as we show in Chapter 3) through countertransference identifying with the client. In each case, the motive of helping the client is the same, but the use of self is very different.

Tabula rasa: countertransference as a barrier to therapy

If we pursue the image of ensuring the therapist as technically honed during training, another aspect associated with this metaphor might be ensuring the aseptic milieu of the laboratory – and since psychotherapy has been called a 'living laboratory', this is perhaps not too far-fetched an image. The initial concern about countertransference – a term that we describe more fully below – might be understood as trying to render the therapist as pure as possible, so that no corrupting and prejudiced feelings and ideas at work in the therapist either interfere with the process of therapy or hinder the objective perception of the patient. Indeed, Freud (1912b: 116) recommended a training analysis as a form of 'psycho-analytic purification'. Just as psychoanalysis developed the idea of the analyst as a blank screen, upon which (or upon whom) projections might be made and transference of past and significant figures might be superimposed, so we might describe the efforts to reduce countertransference in the analyst as the attempt to remove as much of the therapist's 'self' as possible. In effect, the analyst is left as a thinker – a true *analyst* – untroubled by emotions or unconscious thoughts that would otherwise interfere with the 'pure gold of analysis' (Freud 1919: 168). We might currently see this as only one half of the self as engaged with the client: simplistically expressed, as mind more than spirit, or ego rather than the whole self. But the idea behind our expression *tabula rasa* – a clean slate – is one with which some therapists of other persuasions might also in certain respects concur, inasmuch as the therapist is required to enter each new therapeutic encounter without the bias of earlier experience and without theories clouding open attention to what the client describes. We can imagine Rogers, for example, agreeing with Bion's requirement on the therapist to enter the session 'without memory or desire' (Bion 1970). And though we describe in this section the early perceptions of the problem of countertransference, the next chapter illustrates the development of the concept to include a much more therapeutic and positive gloss on the term. In any case, the original intention – to remove as far as possible extraneous elements that are nothing to do with the client – remains just as valid as it ever was.

The term 'countertransference' (sometimes spelled with a hyphen, sometimes without) includes many features. It is in origin a psycho-analytic term, although it has entered the currency of a number of other therapeutic approaches. First used by Freud in a letter to Jung in 1907, he later described it as arising in the analyst 'as a result of the patient's influence on his unconscious feelings' (Freud 1910), a phrase which has a certain ambiguity, since it is not clear whether the patient plays a purely passive role in this, as an unwitting object of the therapist's desire, or 'projects' such feelings for the analyst to pick up. This same ambiguity is found in the 1907 letter, where Freud writes to the younger Jung, embroiled in a difficult relation-ship with Sabina Spielrein:

> Such experiences, though painful, are necessary and hard to avoid. Without them we cannot really know life and what we are dealing with. I myself have never been taken in quite so badly, but I have come very close to it a number of times and had a *narrow escape* [English in original]. I believe that only grim necessities weighing on my work, and the fact that I was ten years older than yourself when I came to psychoanalysis, have saved me from similar experiences. But no lasting harm is done. They help us to develop the thick skin we need and to domin-ate 'countertransference', which is after all a permanent prob-lem for us; they teach us to displace our own affects to best advantage. They are a *'blessing in disguise'* [English in original].
> (McGuire 1974: 230–1)

Barron and Hoffer (1994: 536–40) speculate that because they were erotic feelings, rather than aggressive or narcissistic, it was more difficult for Freud to pursue the 'blessing' part of the equation, instead of reinforcing the need to overcome countertransference in one of his papers on technique, 'Observations on Transference-Love':

Besides, the experiment of letting oneself go a little way in tender feelings for the patient is not altogether without danger. Our control over ourselves is not so complete that we may not suddenly one day go further than we had intended. In my opinion, therefore, we ought not to give up the neutrality towards the patient, which we have acquired through keeping the countertransference in check.

(Freud 1915: 164)

The two aspects of countertransference that were originally more clearly understood were, therefore, the therapist's own transference reactions to the patient – for example, having erotic dreams about the patient even though the patient had neither consciously nor unconsciously hinted of any such feelings towards the therapist – and the therapist responding to the patient's transference – for example, having those same dreams as a response to unconscious erotic feelings which the patient had for the therapist. Whatever the source, both were potentially dangerous and might suggest the analyst required further analysis. The potentiality for identifying the *patient's* unconscious feelings was at this stage neglected.

Jung, although he had provoked the term from Freud in the first instance, says little about countertransference. Indeed, Fordham (1979), one of the leading Jungian interpreters, writes quite critically of Jung's preference for interaction rather than method and the consequence of this for analytical psychology, where for many years study of the analytic situation was delayed on the assumption that there were no clear patterns in the therapeutic relationship. Jung's support for training analysis arose from different motives; not, as in early psychoanalysis, to remove the barriers to effective work, but rather because the patient could go no further than the analyst had done in her or his own analysis. Although the particular form of countertransference in Jungian practice (particularly in the developmental school; see Samuels 1985) has been more open to what it says about the unconscious interaction between analyst and patient, Fordham distinguishes a particular type of countertransference that is similar to the early and classical psychoanalytic use of the term: he calls it 'illusory counter-transference' (Fordham 1969), intending the term to mean that it says nothing about the patient, only about the therapist, whereas 'syntonic counter-transference' is indicative of the therapeutic interaction. Matters become a little complicated when, in a later book, Fordham (1979) refers to 'countertransference' and 'interactional dialectic' as the two distinctions.

The ambiguities of the term clearly vex many of those who write about it. Simplistically, we might distinguish between a form of countertransference that belongs to the therapist alone, and which could interfere with the therapy, and a form of countertransference that has its origins either in the client or in the therapist, or in the interaction between the two, which might be valuable in the therapeutic process. Table 2.1 illustrates just what diverse terms have been used to try and identify these two forms.

Table 2.1 Descriptions of countertransference

Potentially interfering with therapy	Potentially valuable to therapy	Source
Countertransference		Freud (1910)
All of therapist's conscious and unconscious attitudes to patients		Balint and Balint (1939)
Abnormal countertransference	Objective countertransference	Winnicott (1947)
Transferences by analyst to patient		Reich (1951)
Specific reactions to client's transference		Gitelson (1952)
Therapist's transference	Therapist's countertransference	Hoffer (1956)
Neurotic countertransference	Non-neurotic countertransference	Racker (1968)
Complementary countertransference		
	Concordant countertransference	
Illusory countertransference	Syntonic countertransference	Fordham (1969)
Countertransference	Interactional dialectic	Fordham (1979)
	Reflective countertransference Embodied countertransference	Samuels (1993)
Pro-active countertransference	Reactive countertransference	Clarkson (1995)

We shall return to the right-hand side of Table 2.1 in Chapter 3. Here we note not only the variety of terms that express that part of the therapist's self, which it is felt should not interfere with the therapeutic process. We also note that two of the phrases straddle the columns – Balint and Balint (1939) describe how 'the analytical situation is the result of an interplay between the patient's transference and the analyst's counter-transference, complicated by the reactions released in each by the other's transference on to him'; and Racker (1968), who, although making clear distinctions between neurotic and non-neurotic countertransference, also describes two types of countertransference. One of these, complementary countertransference, ranges from being a potential hazard to a potentially valuable tool in analysis. Complementary countertransference is when a therapist reacts in a way that feels foreign, connected in some manner with the patient: the therapist might feel or behave like a figure in the patient's inner world – mother or father perhaps, when either of those parents was also depressed. How this is 'managed' in the therapy itself clearly has implications for whether it is helpful or harmful for the patient.

One of us (Rowan 1998a) has usefully identified various forms of the countertransference that are unlikely to be in the client's interest. This is not to assume that countertransference is just a problem to be overcome, but these are some of the aspects to look for:

- *Defensive* countertransference, when the client triggers off the therapist's unresolved struggles involving dependency, sexuality or aggression.
- *Aim attachment* countertransference, involving unconscious needs such as for success, power, money, love, admiration, voyeurism or guilt, which can distort the therapeutic relationship.
- *Transferential* countertransference, as when the therapist responds as though the client is a parental or sibling figure.
- *Reactive* countertransference, as when the therapist responds to transference distortions as if they were real.
- *Induced* countertransference, as when the therapist takes on a role suggested by the client's needs, such as giving advice.
- *Identification* countertransference, as when the therapist over-identifies with the client or the client's 'child'.
- *Displaced* countertransference, as when the therapist displaces feelings from his or her own personal life on to a client, or when feelings towards one client are displaced and acted out on another.

Identifying these distortions in practice, and countering them, comes about more readily through training, especially the therapist's own therapy and supervision. We examine the way training and supervision are viewed and their relation to the therapist's use of self in Chapter 5.

As Rowan points out, countertransference has generally been underestimated by humanistic therapists. It is our impression that this particular aspect of difficulties in the therapist, which might *adversely* affect the therapy or the therapeutic relationship, appear to be comparatively neglected by the person-centred model and by cognitive and behavioural therapies, inasmuch as references to issues in the therapist are assumed to have been part of their own personal growth process, or to have been covered in training. Person-centred books devote much attention to the positive personal qualities necessary in the therapist, but much less to what blocks progress – although Mearns and Thorne recognize that accepting a client unconditionally may be difficult in some circumstances, and observe that supervision in the person-centred approach 'involves a high degree of personal therapy which is concerned with uncovering and understanding basic needs and fears in the counsellor which might channel her into conditionality' (Mearns and Thorne 1988: 73). But Trower *et al.* (1988), in a basic book on cognitive-behavioural counselling, while devoting a chapter to overcoming blocks to change, solely refer to the client and never to any blocks in the therapist. Nevertheless, as Grant and Crawley (2002: ch. 5) make clear in the companion volume on *Transference and Projection*, cognitive-behavioural therapy shows signs of moving towards greater recognition of the value of blocks in the therapeutic relationship as a way of understanding how these reflect blocks (or schemas) in the client's cognitions and behaviours outside therapy. We might, therefore, anticipate that the significance of the therapeutic relationship in that orientation could in time lead to more focus on blocks in the therapist as well.

The first level of empathy

Although person-centred therapy and, by extension, much humanistic therapy, stresses the positive use of the self by therapists through their empathy, unconditional positive regard and congruence, we suggest that there may be three different levels of empathy, which are related to our own model of the instrumental, the authentic and

Table 2.2 Types of empathy

Category	Column 1 empathy (Chapter 2)	Column 2 empathy (Chapter 3)	Column 3 empathy (Chapter 4)
Self (Rowan)	Mental Ego	Real Self	Soul
Self (Wilber)	Persona/Shadow	Centaur	Psychic/Subtle
Type of boundary	Tight	Loose	Let go
The self is . . .	Defended	Vulnerable	Open to other
Therapist 'label'	Expert at empathy	Wounded Healer	Alter Ego
Aim of therapy	Helping client	Liberation	Communion
Slogan	'I am with you'	'I am open to you'	'I am you'
Analytic	Yes	Yes	Yes
Humanistic	Yes	Yes	Yes
Jungian	No	Yes	Yes
Cognitive-behavioural	Yes	No	No
Family	Yes	Yes	No

the transpersonal, which we deal with respectively in this and the following two chapters.

Hart (1999) has distinguished three phases of empathy, which develop in line with the range and differentiation of a person's feeling capacity. He cites Hoffman: 'One becomes aware that other people's feelings may differ from one's own and are based on their own needs and interpretation of events' (Hoffman 1990: 155). The first phase we depict in Table 2.2, which might be described (as do Mahrer *et al.* 1994) as 'external empathy', where the therapist recognizes what the client is experiencing but remains outside the experience of the other. We have already referred to Rogers' description of empathy as 'as if', where to lose such a state is to become over-identified with the other. Hart (1999) refers both to the self psychologist Kohut and the object relations psychoanalyst Guntrip in this context: Kohut (1984) suggests that empathy is a type of 'vicarious introspection' in which we 'think and feel [ourselves] into the inner life of another person' (p. 82), something we can do because we draw on 'the storehouse of images and memories that we have acquired through . . . our own introspection' (Kohut 1980b: 458). Guntrip (1968: 370–1) writes similarly that 'our understanding is an inference based on our knowledge of ourselves'. As Hart (1999) puts it, 'I know the other through comparing what I understand of their experiences to memories of my own experiences, a logical inference and extrapolation'. He cites Kohn, that this kind of empathy, while 'safe and reasonable', may be limited; and that 'there is real danger that one's cognitive and imaginative capacities will become so sophisticated that one has ceased sharing the experiences of real people' (Kohn 1990: 119).

We suggest that this is 'Column 1 empathy' and belongs in this chapter together with the other technical skills to which we have referred. This is the kind of empathy that can be taught on training courses as a skill. It can be measured on scales of empathy. It is relatively 'safe', in the sense that the therapist is not going to be pulled in too deep. The therapist is defended against undue emotional involvement or pain. It could perhaps be described as 'limited liability' empathy.

Neutrality and abstinence

It is with psychoanalytic practice that neutrality and abstinence are most associated, although most therapies would concur with the need to abstain from sexual contact with the patient, and all would say that it is vital that therapists do not exploit clients for their own ends – in that sense, abstinence may not be so much of an issue. But in psychoanalytic practice, the two terms are virtually co-terminous and are currently under question.

Freud promoted the neutrality of the analyst for a number of good reasons, although perhaps also through fear of the potential damage that can be caused by countertransference. 'Usually, Freud adopted a technical device for personal or practical reasons and only later formulated its theoretical basis' (Schachter 1994: 709). For example, the abstinence of the analyst was felt to motivate the patient, although in the following we see the interests of the analyst as well:

> I cannot advise my colleagues too urgently to model themselves during psychoanalytic treatment on the surgeon who puts aside all his feelings, even his human sympathy . . . The justification for requiring this emotional coldness in the analyst is that it creates the most advantageous conditions for both parties: for the doctor a desirable protection for his own emotional life and for the patient the largest amount of help that we can give him today.
>
> (Freud 1912b: 115)

This 'help' comes through creating a milieu in which the frustration of the setting replicates the frustrations of childhood, permitting catharsis to take place – although, as Schachter (1994: 709) observes, there is 'an early inconsistency in Freud's views: that while abstinence is the prime motivator for analytic work, love, which is frustrated by abstinence, is also a prime motivator for analytic work'. 'Love is the great educator', wrote Freud (1916: 312).

Neutrality (or the actual word Freud wrote, *indifferenz*) also respects the individuality of the patient: 'The analyst respects the patient's individuality and does not seek to remould him in accordance with his own . . . personal ideals; he is glad to avoid giving advice and instead to arouse the patient's power of initiative' (Freud 1923: 251).

Yet there are in the first three decades of the practice of psychoanalysis a number of examples of the absence of this neutrality in Freud himself, where he appears to show no consciousness of there being countertransference issues. Freud was not averse to disclosing details about his personal and family life, and even gave money to patients in financial difficulty (Obholzer 1980: 33–4, 60–1). Indeed, the picture of the early analysts' neutrality is a confusing one, with records of boundary violations in the initial period of the development of analytic technique, which would today be seen by some purists as anathema, and by most therapists generally as completely inappropriate (e.g. Klein's analysis of her own children). Ferenczi questioned the passivity of the analyst and experimented with what he called 'mutual analysis' (Dupont 1995: xx–xxii), whereby the therapist also discussed his own issues with the patient. Freud criticized his colleague's experiments as a 'third puberty', but Ferenczi in turn criticized Freud's overly impersonal pedagogic technique (Dupont 1995: xv, xxiv). Today, the style of analysts varies so greatly that it is inaccurate to continue to stereotype psychoanalytic therapists as presenting themselves as blank screens; for example, Couch's full description of his analysis with Anne Freud includes the phrase, 'She was always her real self and an analyst at the same time' (Couch 1995: 158).

The experience of being in analysis therefore varies: some patients will have met silent therapists and valued this, others will have been put off by it. The experience of other patients will be of analysts who are relational, while retaining their objectivity in seeking to understand both the client's material and the process of therapy itself. This variation in practice is reflected in the debate in the literature, notably from the 1980s onwards. Schachter describes this as follows:

Modern views of abstinence and neutrality can be ordered along a dimension which, at one extreme, places a great emphasis on the value of both stances, with departures seen as manipulations of the transference [e.g. Shapiro (1984) and Poland (1984)], and, at the other extreme, values the analyst's empathic affirmation of the patient, with abstinence and neutrality viewed as damaging because they are experienced by the patient as critical acts by an aloof analyst [e.g. self psychologists such as Bacal (1985) or Tolpin (1988); and constructivists such as Gill (1982) and Hoffman (1992)]. What obfuscates this ordering of views along a single dimension is the dichotomous characterisation of analyst behaviour as either technical or personal (non-technical) . . . In the middle of this scale are the analysts who believe that, irrespective of whether abstinence and neutrality or affirmation are more highly valued, the interaction of emotional forces in patient and analyst profoundly, unwittingly and repeatedly influences the analyst's behaviour, so that neither abstinence and neutrality nor affirmation are seen as choices of the analyst, independent of the patient's experience of the analyst's behaviour.

(Schachter 1994: 713)

The answer to Hoffer's (1985: 772) question, 'Are genuine involvement with another person and honest neutrality somehow antithetical?', appears to be 'no'. We appear to be describing the value of the therapist being able to slip relatively effortlessly between involvement (intersubjectivity) and stepping back in an attempt to understand the possibilities revealed in therapeutic relationship (objectivity).

Conclusion

Page (1999) takes Jung's term 'the shadow' and applies it to the work of the counsellor, as that which is 'unknown' to conscious awareness and which may be harmful. He includes in this the shadow of the counselling profession itself. He quotes Street on the different layers of motivation to become therapists as including 'less palatable factors . . . the need to be needed, a perhaps slightly macabre curiosity that borders on voyeurism, an enjoyment of the sense of being important for our clients' (Page 1999: 12). As we have in this chapter, Page says that counsellors develop a persona for their counselling work, which is really a false self, all the more confusing because it is supposed to express authenticity. The personal shadow lurks behind this persona, but also behind the ego itself. The persona need not, of course, be the same as a false self, since the persona performs a particular function in a particular setting. Only when the persona takes over does it create a false self. But Page's warning is apposite, since what we have been describing in this chapter is one level of the therapist's use of self, which, important though it is, can become too limiting.

We need to reiterate as we move into a second level of the therapist's use of self, that what we have described in this chapter is not purely a negative view of the therapist's use of self. The learned skills, the outward behaviour and the persona of the therapist constitute one aspect of the therapist's work. Countertransference, however it is termed, can have a negative effect and therefore, where possible, needs to be identified. To varying extents, depending on the style of the therapy and perhaps the character of the therapist, neutrality and abstinence have a part to play in promoting the welfare of the client. Similarly, a simple level of empathy such as we have described is the foundation for deeper empathic responses.

Most forms of training address these different elements, providing what we might call a framework, or a container for that other aspect of the therapist's use of self, the way he or she recognizes, uses and understands experiences with clients as an inner process, which may or may not be expressed in external behaviour or in overt phrases. If humanistic therapies have been characterized by greater openness to the therapist's relating with the client, this has perhaps at times been to the neglect of technical implications and some of the potentiality for harm in the therapeutic relationship. And if some other approaches have emphasized the technical, almost role-playing aspect of the therapist, even where the personal development aspect of training has been seen as important, it has taken time for them to recognize the potential in the greater use of the therapist's inner self. It is these further potentialities to which we turn our attention in the next chapter.

CHAPTER 3

The authentic self

It must have been somewhat tongue in cheek that Freud pronounced psychoanalysis, in common with education and government, as an 'impossible profession'. Psychotherapy is certainly a tough one, making demands upon the therapist as well as the client, and proportionately, if not identically, as disturbing for the therapist as it is for the client who is experiencing severe psychological disturbance. In these instances, the risks of damage to both parties are high. No wonder mistakes have been made from the beginning: we think of Breuer fleeing from involvement with Anna O. Strong feelings have led to some therapists being carried away in enthusiasm or in abusive dealings with their clients; and the need for protecting the client (although perhaps just as much, if we are honest, protecting the therapist) has at points in the relatively brief history of the profession possibly led to some inhibition of the very factors which more and more research has shown to be important in therapeutic efficacy. These factors transcend orientation and, although they may go by different names and may take different forms according to the modality we have in mind, it is the willingness of the therapist to be more open to them that is the subject of this chapter. We believe that all therapists who have done sufficient work on themselves can move into this further level of openness and self-awareness.

Shadley's study, originally published in 1987, concludes that 'the manner in which therapists made use of themselves in therapy had less to do with their theoretical stance than with personal realities such as gender, developmental stage, and personal attitudes' (Shadley 2000: 192). There is confirmation in that study of the researcher's premise that the professional self is a constantly evolving system, changed by the conscious and unconscious interplay affecting the clinician. The most important result in the second section of the study was that therapists from all orientations found genuineness to be one of the most important qualities for the effective use of self. That genuineness may again go under different names. We provide in this chapter sufficient explanation for the reader to consider how genuineness, congruence, empathy, intuition, authenticity and the ability to fully use the countertransference and projective identification (such being some of the terms different modalities use) might or might not be related.

In the previous chapter, we showed how different modalities approach the question of the interference of the therapist in the therapeutic process. It is, as it were, the negative side of the therapist's self, which needs to be monitored, so as not to prejudice the therapy, not to misinform the therapist or misunderstand the client. The danger is that over-concern with interference of the self might lead to unhelpful abstinence or even the development of a false self in the therapist – perhaps like Winnicott's (1965: 140–52) use of the term, a false self built upon *compliance* with what is taught in training. In this chapter, it is the more positive use of the therapist's self that comes into focus: what Winnicott called the 'true self' and others might call personhood, or the genuine, the authentic or the real self. We look at ways in which the therapist is aware of and uses her or his own emotions, thoughts and reactions in the service of understanding the client, and in creating a relationship that serves the interests of the client. We look at views on what the therapist might choose to disclose of these reactions, or even what the therapist chooses to disclose in the way of more personal information.

Although we would want to avoid encouraging a false self in the therapist, we stress, as we did earlier, that we are not here suggesting that it is a question of *either* technical skills and tested methods *or* the personal qualities of the therapist; neither do we regard the technical skills and care not to let the self intrude unhelpfully as indicative of an inferior approach, or of necessity a sign of a false presentation of the self. But it is a limited one. We should at the outset lay out our own position, that we would regard the use of self as so far described in this book as limited to relatively short-term or solution-oriented forms of work in therapy, and as likely to be ineffectual in longer-term or more open-ended forms. Nor do we want either to imply that until the 'negative' counter-productive side of the self is mastered, the positive use of self must wait. Those who suggest that it is only with experience that therapists can begin to drop the mask, in our opinion short-change the creative possibilities open to trainees and fledgling therapists, whose personal learning can also be used judiciously in their practice. As Little observes, 'outstanding results' can come in therapy both from

> those experienced analysts who have gone through the stage of over-cautiousness . . . [and from] beginners who are not afraid to allow their unconscious impulses a considerable degree of freedom because, through lack of experience, like children, they do not know or understand the dangers, and do not recognize them. It works out well in quite a high proportion of cases, because the positive feelings preponderate.
>
> (Little 1951: 36–7)

Although personal work in therapy is a very good way of moving from the instrumental to the authentic (from the Mental Ego to the Centaur, in Wilber's terms), it is by no means the only way. Life experience can offer its own challenges and opportunities to foster growth in the personality.

Psychodynamic concepts: extending definitions of countertransference

It was perhaps necessary that the initial identification in psychoanalysis of countertransference was seen as a 'problem', one that needed to be overcome as far as possible in working as a therapist. The same had happened with the concept of transference, initially seen as a barrier, yet later as an essential part in psychoanalytic work for re-living earlier traumatic relationships. Countertransference in psychoanalytic theory was seen originally as an unconscious phenomenon and, by its very nature, what is unconscious is difficult to access, hence the felt need for intensive personal analysis. But this changed, as Tyson (1986: 151) summarizes: '(1) from Ucs to Cs, (2) from reactions to transference to all reactions, (3) from the analyst's neurosis to the analyst's functioning, (4) from self-analysis to self-scrutiny, (5) from obstacle to contribution'. Beyond this several subtle distinctions have been made in mapping the way countertransference functions.

It is the fifth of these changes, 'from obstacle to contribution', that is most relevant to this section. Paula Heimann (1950), a British Kleinian analyst, is normally credited with initiating the view that countertransference should include all the feelings that a therapist experiences with a patient, and that these feelings can be utilized as a resource, providing insight into the patient's unconscious conflicts and defences. The opening words of her short paper succinctly challenge the conventions of the time:

> I have been struck by the widespread belief amongst candidates that the counter-transference is nothing but a source of trouble. Many candidates are afraid and feel guilty when they become aware of feelings towards their patients and consequently aim at avoiding any emotional response and at becoming completely unfeeling and 'detached'.
>
> (Heimann 1950: 81)

This is, of course, exactly what we have suggested is the attitude of the analyst who is stuck at the instrumental level. Heimann admits there are some misreadings of Freud that suggest a detached attitude in the analyst, but prefers to follow Ferenczi who 'not only acknowledges that the analyst has a wide variety of feelings towards his patient, but recommends that he should at times express them openly' (Heimann 1950: 81). We discuss the question of disclosing countertransference and other feelings below.

In fact, Heimann was not the first to raise such questions about countertransference. Hann-Kende had made similar references in 1933, but at that time attracted little attention. Winnicott similarly suggests a different way of regarding countertransference in his paper, 'On hate in the countertransference', first delivered in 1947. There he distinguishes 'objective counter-transference, or . . . the analyst's love and hate in reaction to the actual personality and behaviour of the patient, based on objective observation' (Winnicott 1975: 195). Little (1951) similarly treats countertransference from several different perspectives, which she says are difficult to disentangle, and she refers in passing to the value of revealing countertransference feelings to the patient. Khan (1974), a colleague of Winnicott's, describes countertransference as 'a clinical instrument of perception' (p. 68), based on 'the conscious and total sensitivity of the analyst towards the patient' (p. 137) and on the 'non-pathological capacity of the analyst's affectivity, intelligence, and imagination to comprehend the total reality of the patient' (p. 206). This now describes well the authentic attitude we are trying to convey in this chapter. Even earlier, but probably unknown to these psychoanalytic writers, Jung had emphasized the need for the analyst to be influenced by the patient unconsciously; he refers to this as 'counter-transference evoked by the transference'. This was first published in English in 1933 (Jung 1966: para. 163).

Discussions about countertransference in psychoanalytic literature have continued for more than half a century, with an excellent summary of the concept as used in the past and at the turn of the twentieth century in an article by Theodore Jacobs (1999: 575–94). Rather than go into detail about the debate itself, we here select a number of the key terms that have been used, which in most cases express the value of exploring the emotional reactions and intuitive responses of the therapist towards the patient (see Table 2.1).

Taking the references in the second column of Table 2.1 ('potentially valuable to therapy') in chronological order, we have referred already to Winnicott's term 'objective countertransference', which appears in his 1947 paper 'Hate in the countertransference' (Winnicott 1975: 194–203). There Winnicott specifically refers to the need to contain both the hatred in the therapist and the hatred in the patient, until such a point as it may be spoken about: 'the analyst must be prepared to bear strain without expecting the patient to know anything about what he is doing, perhaps over a long period of time' (p. 198). He is referring here to the therapist's 'own fear and hate' (p. 198), which is to be distinguished from the more usual modern view of countertransference – namely, that it is a reaction to the patient's transference and, as such, is informative of as yet unconscious feelings and the style of relating in the patient. This latter view is the meaning of such terms as Hoffer's (1956) 'therapist's countertransference' or Clarkson's (1995) 'reactive countertransference'. Clarkson draws upon Lewin's (1963) terms 'proactive' and 'reactive' to designate whether the subject (i.e. the therapist) originates the stimulus (proacts) or responds to (reacts) to a stimulus from the other (i.e. the patient): 'This differentiation separates two major kinds of countertransference depending on whether the psychotherapist is reacting to a patient or proactively introducing his or her own transference into the psychotherapeutic relationship' (Clarkson 1995: 89).

But it is important to note that Winnicott went back on his bold 1947 thinking in a later paper originally written in 1960, where he prefers the original use of 'counter-transference' (as he then calls it, with a hyphen) and where he distinguishes 'reactions' from countertransference, citing the example of when he got hit by a patient: she 'got a little bit of the real me . . . but a reaction is not counter-transference' (Winnicott 1965: 164). This reminds us that we are concerned in this chapter not just with what the client appears to 'make' the therapist feel, but with how the therapist uses all of his or her cognitive, emotional and intuitive responses, whatever their origin.

Winnicott's 1947 paper is to be preferred to his 1960 paper, a somewhat tetchy response to the Jungian Michael Fordham (see below). In the earlier paper, he refers to another aspect of countertransference which is valuable: he distinguishes between abnormal feelings in the analyst that show the need for more personal analysis, and identification with the patient from the analyst's own experience and development. The latter provides a unique and positive aspect to the analyst's work, making each analyst different from any other analyst. So one person's countertransference will be different from another's, and the patient may be helped because a particular analyst can identify with a particular aspect of them, which another analyst cannot. Such an idea recognizes the individual personality of each therapist and that one therapist may be the right person for some clients but not for others, because of the ability or inability to identify fully with a particular client, not from training or lack of it, but from personal character and personal experience.

Sandler *et al.* (1973) make the point that the use of the word 'counter' in English can either be 'alongside' or 'against' – 'counterpart' means something complementary, 'counteract' means to act against. This ambiguity of the term in compound words may help to explain the different uses to which countertransference has been put in analytic terminology; but it also supports the potential for complementarity in the way the therapist uses this part of her or his experience. Complementary countertransference is a term used by Racker (1968) and by Clarkson (1995), the latter also borrowing Racker's term 'concordant countertransference'. At first sight, 'complementary' and 'concordant' look like synonyms, but each is used somewhat differently by each author to describe ways in which the therapist is drawn into the therapeutic relationship.

Racker (1957), who originally wrote a paper distinguishing these two types of relationship towards the patient, starts with the proposition that, in therapy, 'everything happens that can happen in one personality faced with another' (p. 311). The predominating tendency in the therapist is the attempt to understand, but alongside this 'there exist toward the patient virtually all the other possible tendencies, fears, and other feelings that one person may have toward another' (p. 311). Wishing to understand predisposes the therapist to identify with the patient, since it is this that promotes comprehension.

> The analyst may achieve this aim by identifying . . . each part of
> his personality with the corresponding psychological part in the
> patient – his id with the patient's id, his ego with the ego, his
> superego with the superego, accepting these identifications in his
> consciousness . . . recognition of what belongs to another as one's
> own ('his part of you is I') and on the equation of what is one's
> own with what belongs to another ('this part of me is you').
>
> (Racker 1957: 311–12)

This is what Racker calls concordant countertransference, and which
he identifies as 'non-neurotic countertransference'.

'But', he goes on, 'this does not always happen, nor is it all that
happens' (Racker 1957: 311). If the therapist has difficulty identifying with the patient, then complementary identifications take place,
where the therapist begins to feel treated like that part of the patient
with which the therapist has been unable to identify. For example,
if the therapist is unable to identify with the patient's aggressiveness, due to a difficulty in the therapist acknowledging his or her
own aggressive tendencies, the patient's aggressiveness is rejected;
the therapist may then feel like one of the rejecting figures in the
patient's internal world (and past history) towards whom the patient's
aggression is directed. Yet, by being attuned to this complementary
countertransference, the therapist may be able to identify what he
or she does not understand, which may in turn lead the therapist
to the more valuable concordant countertransference. That is the
reason in Table 2.1 for placing complementary countertransference
across the two columns, 'potentially interfering' and 'potentially
valuable'.

In *The Political Psyche*, Samuels (1993), a post-Jungian analyst, uses
two different terms, 'reflective countertransference' and 'embodied
countertransference', which in their functioning appear similar to
Racker's use of the adjectives 'concordant' and 'complementary'.
Samuels' example is that an analyst may feel depressed after seeing a
patient, but this may be the result of identifying with the patient's
unconscious depression – something that might be able to be used
in empathic responses in later sessions. But an analyst may react or
behave in a way that feels foreign to him or her, yet still be connected in some manner with the patient: the therapist might feel or
behave like a figure in the patient's inner world, mother or father
perhaps, when either of those parents was depressed. In this instance,
instead of being depressed as the patient may unconsciously feel
(concordant or reflective countertransference), the analyst becomes

like the depressed parent the patient once had (embodied counter-transference). This is also in a fashion complementary, although not in this case, as Racker suggests, because the analyst has some difficulty identifying with depressed feelings. We examine a slightly different meaning of 'embodied' countertransference below.

Concordant transference is probably also to be equated with what the Jungian analyst Michael Fordham (1969) calls 'syntonic counter-transference', where the analyst's feelings and behaviour are in tune with, a counterpart to, the patient's inner world. In 1979, Fordham uses a different term, 'interactional dialectic', by which he refers to a constant interplay between the projections and introjections of the patient and the analyst. This is almost identical to Racker's notion that:

> every transference situation provokes a counter-transference situation, which arises out of the analyst's identification of himself with the analysand's (internal) objects. These counter-transference situations may be repressed or emotionally blocked, but probably cannot be avoided: certainly they should not be avoided if full understanding is to be achieved.
>
> (Racker 1968: 137)

An example that Fordham provides may be helpful. He describes working with a female patient whose sessions were preoccupied with what was going on inside the analyst, and her conviction that she was accurate in her perceptions. She interspersed these assertions with questions to the analyst. Fordham says there were obvious reasons for not answering the questions, but he refrained from doing so for another reason – because he was convinced that to do so would be a blunder. He did not know where this feeling came from, and he held back from making any interpretation based upon his feeling of what was going on, until one day the patient was talking about her father and how *he* did not answer her questions. Fordham could then see how this relationship was being re-enacted in the transference, and how a possible interpretation could be: 'Now I see why I don't answer your questions; it is as it was with your father. You made me like your father by the very persistence of your questions, to which you did not expect an answer'.

What he also stresses is that countertransference interpretations are based upon affective processes rather than on intellectual processes (Fordham *et al.* 1974: 247–9). Racker gives an example of complementary countertransference that has some similarities to

Fordham's example, in that it is set off by what Racker calls a 'spontaneous thought' in the therapist. (We note Fordham's 'feeling' and Racker's 'thought': does this suggest Jungian analysts work more from their feelings, while psychoanalytic therapists work more from their thinking?) In Racker's vignette, a woman patient asked her therapist whether it was true that another analyst had separated from his wife and remarried. The idea (again note that it is an *idea* here more than a *feeling* as it was in Fordham) occurred to the therapist that the patient would really like to know whether this other analyst had married one of his *patients*. He then supposed that the patient was wondering whether he too might separate from his wife and marry her. Avoiding making any suggestion to this effect, the therapist returned to his initial thought and asked whether the patient was thinking about the analyst's second wife. She laughed and said, 'Yes I was wondering whether she was not one of his patients'. What Racker also notes here is that the therapist did not block his own feelings towards his patient by repressing them as unsavoury. He was able to use them to understand more about the woman's feelings towards him.

Clarkson (1995: 90–1), an integrative psychotherapist, drawing in the main upon different strands of psychoanalytic theory, combines her distinction between proactive and reactive countertransference with the terms 'complementary' and 'concordant', thereby defining four types of countertransference. Reactive countertransference, to recapitulate, is the response of the therapist induced in the therapist by the patient. Proactive countertransference is used for feelings coming primarily from the therapist. The four types of countertransference outlined by Clarkson (1995: 91–2) are:

- *Complementary reactive countertransference*: the therapist feels, thinks and is tempted to behave in a way that would 'be complementary to the real or fantasised projection of the patient's historical past selves'.
- *Concordant reactive countertransference*: 'a literal emotional attunement to an affective or feeling state which is problematical or painful to the client'.
- *Complementary proactive countertransference*: 'the psychotherapist complements the client's real or fantasised projection as the caretaker or child of the psychotherapist's own past' projected on to the client.
- *Concordant proactive countertransference*: 'the therapist imagines they are attending to the client's experience, but in fact they are

replicating their own past . . . a kind of identification' – or again, we might add, the therapist's projection on to the client.

From this it would appear that reactive countertransference is a type of introjection by the therapist from the client, enabling the therapist to identify with the client or with figures from the client's past; and that proactive countertransference, that aspect of the self which Chapter 2 has concentrated upon, is a type of projection by the therapist on to the client.

Michael Fordham was one of the leading Jungian writers in Britain in the third quarter of the twentieth century. There appears to be a characteristic difference between the Jungian and the psycho-analytic valuation of countertransference, because although Fordham refers to 'illusory countertransference' as descriptive of the analyst's own responses, mistakenly understood to come from the patient, he does not put such a negative gloss on this phenomenon, as some Freudians or Kleinians have done in defining what we might call classical countertransference. Fordham does not want to pathologize countertransference. This reflects the more positive view that Jungians generally have of the unconscious, as being more than a repository for what is repressed: it is rather a storehouse of those aspects that are essential for psychological growth. There is potentiality for learning from illusory countertransference: it is a means of increasing the self-knowledge of the analyst, thereby enabling identification to become more accurate. We have already noted above that Racker similarly suggests that complementary countertransference can shift from being unhelpful to being potentially valuable as concordant countertransference.

In his later writing, Fordham (1979) questions whether it is any longer appropriate to refer to the interactions of analysis from the analyst's side as countertransference – it is a normal part of the analysis. This is not quite the same as Winnicott's assertion that reactions are not countertransference, since Fordham seems to assert the identity between the two, whereas Winnicott completely distinguishes them. Fordham's view of the interactional element in therapy may be further illustrated by a reference in Samuels (1985: 122) to some research into countertransference by four analytical psychologists in Germany. They sum up their findings by the exclamation of one of their group that 'the patients continually say what I am thinking and feeling at the moment' – in other words, not only does the therapist pick up and feed back to the patient feelings and thoughts that the patient recognizes, but (and this must be a familiar experience to many therapists) just as the therapist is formulating an idea in his or her own mind, the patient says it first. Where do such feelings and thoughts start? In the therapist? Or in the patient? Or in them both simultaneously in response to some other event external or internal to the therapy? Who knows! But the term that Fordham uses to distinguish this part of the therapeutic relationship, 'interactional dialectic', like Stolorow and Atwood's (1992) term 'intersubjectivity', expresses it well.

What becomes clear is that making hard and fast distinctions between proactive and reactive, illusory and syntonic, positive and negative, complementary and concordant is unwise. Although Clarkson (1995) represents the views of many analysts that 'it is essential that the clinician be able to separate out proactive from reactive countertransference' (p. 92), it is, as she points out, rarely as neat as that. What starts as complementary can become concordant, what starts as illusory can lead to syntonic countertransference, and vice versa: what starts as reactive countertransference can give rise to proactive countertransference. Clarkson cites an example from the Kohutian self-psychologist Wolf, that a therapist may recognize in his or her countertransference feelings how a patient wants the therapist to be such an ideal figure, in order for the patient to feel good by basking in the reflection of this idealized person. But a patient's idealization may, in turn, make some therapists feel grandiose ('I am so important to this patient, I am the only one who can love them'), which can lead to therapist abuse; or make others too uncomfortable with the huge expectations put upon them ('I can never do enough for this patient'), leading to self-depreciation in the therapist, which is anti-therapeutic for both parties (Wolf 1988: 144). These are, of course, unreconstructed ego reactions, which belong to the instrumental approach (Chapter 2), rather than to the authentic approach we are considering in the present chapter.

Racker (1968) gives a similar example: a male therapist becomes aware through countertransference that he is experienced by a female client as being a 'thieving analyst', and that this is a defensive projection of the client's own greediness. But the therapist on an emotional level feels resentment at the client because she reminds him of his own robbing mother, and so he is rendered useless as an analyst. Only if he works through his neurotic countertransference can he turn the feelings into a complementary countertransference, which will then permit him to work on this aspect in the client.

These examples of the way in which one type of countertransference can turn into another might also be framed as how easily the two can be confused. Given that underlying all psychodynamic thinking there lies the notion that the unconscious is in essence unknowable, how can we ever really know what is, for example, proactive and what is reactive? Samuels (1993: 45–6) highlights some important questions that need to be raised given the current psychoanalytic understanding of countertransference, and the current acceptance that it is in the main an invaluable tool in therapy. He refers to five areas that give cause for concern:

1 How can the therapist actually tell whether what is believed through a countertransference reaction to be a communication from the patient is a genuine communication and not an unresolved issue in the therapist?
2 Is there not a risk that, by treating countertransference reactions as communications from the patient, the patient is made responsible for everything?
3 Does not the idea that the therapist can pick up what the patient is communicating through countertransference feed the patient's fantasy of the magical omniscience of the therapist, and the persecutory anxiety that the therapist can penetrate the patient's mind?
4 Use of the countertransference may lead to therapist self-disclosure more often than one would expect in a more classical neutrality stance. Is it always good to reveal what you feel as a therapist? We return to this question below.
5 Given that there is so much possibility of confusion and, indeed, that some would say that this confusion is part of the interactional process between therapist and client, does this not espouse confusion, whereas therapy should be about making things clearer?

Embodied countertransference

We have referred above to Samuels' term 'embodied countertransference', where he appears to use the adjective metaphorically, so that psychologically the therapist embodies some significant person in the patient's inner world. But he also refers to physical reactions in the therapist as part of this embodiment, so that feelings are literally embodied. He gives an example:

After the memories came, she was very angry with me indeed. One session, she got up and sat in the desk chair which is located behind my usual chair . . . She told me what she would like to do to my head with an instrument, and this became an expressed fantasy of what she was doing . . . But I was not frightened. In fact I had the most pleasant, warm sensation in my lower legs and feet, as if seated before a fire. I went on to have a vision of a small and comfortable living-room in which we were both sitting. In my mind's ear I could hear the rustle of 'my' newspaper. I was smoking my pipe anyway. I said: 'You're watching daddy read his paper. It's pleasant. Part of you wants it to go on for ever. Part of you wants him to look up and acknowledge you. The tension is what is making you angry. You're smashing my brains up because that settles the question of whether I'll notice you of my own accord'. For the first time, she and I could grasp the telos of her exceedingly dramatic and demanding behaviour . . . I had experienced an embodied countertransference.

(Samuels 1989: 81)

This particular term 'embodied', which Samuels uses, emphasizes that countertransference can be experienced in a physical way and not just in spontaneous thoughts or psychological feelings. Clarkson (1995), too, reminds us that 'transference and countertransference phenomena are carried across not only in a verbal content but also in non-verbal ways through body language, smells, or atmospheric and contextual cues' (p. 90). Orbach (1995) also explores the idea in an article on 'Countertransference and the false self'. First, she extends Winnicott's concept of the false self, particularly when understanding eating disorders, to the false body and the bodily sense in some women that is 'both real and unreal'. It is as if some women have constructed a false body in which they live, and they search by some means or other for a true body. Orbach then takes this idea and discusses bodily reactions in the therapist: how reflecting upon her own body in the consulting room has led to her understanding a patient's view of the patient's own body. Orbach cites as one example a patient whose hatred of her own body was a constant feature of the analysis. Orbach saw this as a step towards the patient's recognition that she had a defensively constructed difficult, false body, which had to be acknowledged as such if she were to find something of her true body. Simultaneously, Orbach had what she describes as 'the experience of becoming deeply and comfortably into awareness of my own body and how very at ease I felt with it'. It was as if her patient had created for herself, via her therapist, 'a good wholesome, nourishing and stable contented body . . . the (external) body object that she needed in order to struggle through to finding a body for herself' (Orbach 1995: 9). Orbach shared this experience with the patient and showed her how a woman who was normally so destructive had been able to create in the session a 'perfect body' in the therapist (see also Ross (2000) on somatic countertransference).

Winnicott makes a curious reference to physical reactions, as though he both values them and yet puts them to one side. After saying that he is not an intellectual, he writes that he works 'very much from the body-ego', but that he thinks of himself 'working with easy but conscious mental effort. Ideas and feelings come to mind' (Winnicott 1965: 161). But then he says that 'I may have stomach ache but this does not usually affect my interpretations; and on the other hand I may have been somewhat stimulated erotic-ally or aggressively by an idea given by the patient, but again this does not usually affect my interpretative work' (pp. 161–2). Here we see the remarkably intuitive Winnicott having to restrain himself, at least in print, even though obviously aware of his bodily responses to the patient.

Projective identification

The question arises whether the view of countertransference that has come to predominate in analytic circles is related to other con-cepts referred to elsewhere in psychoanalytic terminology, such as projective identification, intuition and empathy (particularly in Kohut's self-psychology); and to other concepts that are accorded special significance in humanistic therapies, again such as empathy and intuition, as well as variously congruence, genuineness, reson-ance and presence, all of which represent descriptions of the therapist as needing to be fully in touch with herself or himself, as well as fully relating to the client. In the sections that follow, we examine the way these terms are understood in different modalities and whether they are related.

Projective identification, like transference and countertransference, originates in psychoanalytic theory and, like those allied terms, is accorded huge significance in understanding the therapeutic rela-tionship. Rowan (1998a) remarks that just as countertransference was once regarded as wholly negative, but was then seen as a valu-able indicator of what is really going on, much the same shift has happened with regard to projective identification. At first it was viewed as a purely negative and quite rare phenomenon in borderline cases, but it came to be seen as an important key to the whole interpersonal process. But Rowan also notes that, in the humanistic tradition, there is some suspicion of these phenomena, as if they obscure authentic interaction, which is central to the humanistic method and aim. The therapist is still in touch with her or his inner responses, but this is a conscious process and is called 'genuineness'.

In projective identification, the therapist experiences feelings that are strange and alien and that do not appear to belong to the therapist. He or she is feeling something that the client is not prepared to feel and instead unconsciously projects into (not just onto) the therapist. Rowan (1998a) cites an example that has some similarities to Orbach's embodied countertransference and contrasts with Winnicott's attitude to his stomach ache!

> I recall listening to a graduate intern's report of his clinical progress and noting how relaxed and clear he appeared to be. Everything seemed in order. I began to suffer a terrible stomach ache. I supposed the problem was mine, something I'd eaten or some piece of my own personal work. I decided to tell my supervisee that I had a stomach ache that had come on suddenly. I asked him if he was sitting on something he wasn't talking about. He thought for a moment, then stared at me, then burst into tears. My stomach ache began to abate. There was in fact a terrible piece of business going on in his life that he had tucked away so carefully that in coming into my office he'd forgotten it for the time being.
>
> (Baldwin 1997: 95)

Rowan observes that, while containing such feelings, the experience needs to be shared, if not always directly; although in this example the supervisor does refer explicitly to the stomach ache, but not suggesting it was to do with the supervision. Sharing is in line with the humanistic emphasis on openness and self-disclosure. We discuss this question more fully below.

The idea of projective identification comes originally from the Kleinian School and is well described by Hinshelwood (1989). It is also considered alongside transference and projection in the companion volume in this series by Grant and Crawley (2002). It has become a popular concept, perhaps over-popular inasmuch as it has become one of those catch-all phrases that may be used to explain anything the therapist experiences.

Rowan (1998a: 133) distinguishes countertransference as belonging to the therapist and projective identification as coming from the client. Here is yet another way of attempting to disentangle what starts where. Britton (1998: 5–6) distinguishes between *acquisitive* projective identification and *attributive* projective identification: the former is a delusional state, such as when someone believes they are Napoleon; the latter, which comes from Bion's (1962: 31) extension of the concept and is the type which we are considering here, is when an aspect of the self is attributed to another person, which may induce change in the other, making them take in and in some sense 'become' the projection. In practical terms, Bion's theory supports the view of the therapist as a container for the patient's unwanted thoughts and feelings, which can in time be returned safely to the patient.

The precise relationship between projection, projective identification and countertransference has been the subject of considerable debate in psychoanalytic circles, made more confusing when some of those participating in it have not fully understood the Kleinian distinctions between projection and projective identification. This is not the place to document the debate (but see Grotstein 1994). We may note, however, that the American analyst Grotstein (1994: 583) believes that 'the concept of counter-transference has become too all-inclusive and does not distinguish between psychopathology and normal conditions'. He writes:

> The analytic instrument that the analyst uses, i.e., his mind, comprises the employment of intuition, introspection, empathic observation, and emotional resonance à la Stanislavsky with similar situations within him-/herself that correspond to the emotional material produced by the patient. In other words, I believe these are the normal components of the thinking repertoire of the analyst's psychoanalytic instrumentation.
>
> (Grotstein 1994: 582–3)

Grotstein (1994) observes that the current view of countertransference – that is, the therapist's 'way of being emotionally responsive in meaningful ways to the patient's material' (p. 583) – means that thought is the 'analytic instrument'. Note here once more the psychoanalytic bias towards 'mind', which appears to subsume feelings ('emotional resonance').

Grotstein prefers a different term to projective identification:

> I think the more appropriate term is that proffered by Money-Kyrle (1956), the analyst's introjective identification. Furthermore, it is important to distinguish between partial introjective identification and total, the latter being totally unconscious and hypnotically controlling or possessive of the analyst, whereas partial introjective identification connotes that the analyst's observing ego is able to perceive an idiosyncratic experience that is worthy of clinical note. In other words, the analyst's total introjective identificatory response to his/her patient's projective identifications would amount to a folie à deux, a non-therapeutic collusion, a mutual resistance, whereas partial or trial introjective identification allows the analyst's observing ego to use his very emotional experience of his patient's projections as an analytic instrument.
>
> (Grotstein 1994: 583)

What is valuable here is the reminder that therapists, while letting themselves become immersed in the inner world of the patient, need to preserve an observing part of the self, which monitors and processes what is happening to and in the therapist. Grotstein also usefully identifies a further aspect of countertransference:

> that of the analyst's emotional response to having responded emotionally, that is, how (s)he feels about having been influenced in this way. Analysts may get frightened, angry, depressed, saddened, disappointed, upset, etc., because of the very fact that their psychical/emotional system has been penetrated by their experience with the patient.
>
> (Grotstein 1994: 584)

This is a necessary reminder that, in addition to feeling 'for the patient', therapists have their own feelings to consider and will inevitably need their own support to go on containing the strong emotions and fearsome thoughts that they carry for their patients. Grotstein's image of the therapist and patient is that of the Pieta: Mary holding the tortured Christ figure. Of course, this more sophisticated use of introjected identification is peculiar to the authentic stage of development. At the instrumental stage, emotions do indeed take over 'when they think they will' and we get total introjected identification rather than partial or trial identification. This is why anyone working in this area has to take personal therapy so seriously.

Carl Rogers, who from a person-centred perspective strongly objected to the term 'countertransference', might nonetheless be seen
as supporting some of these ideas. In an interview with Michele
Baldwin, he says:

> To be a fully authentic therapist, I think that you have to feel
> entirely secure as a person. This allows you to let go of yourself,
> knowing confidently that you can come back . . . I think it is
> important to realise that one has a need and a right to preserve
> and protect oneself. A therapist has a right to give, but not to
> get worn out trying to be giving.
>
> (Baldwin 2000: 36, 31)

The concept of projective identification or introjected identification adds to our understanding of the way in which the self of the
therapist is open to be used by the patient. Several analysts point
to the way in which the therapist needs to be used by the patient.
Grotstein (1994) is one; Bollas is another:

> For differing reasons and in various ways, analysands re-create
> their infantile life in the transference in such a determined and
> unconsciously accomplished way that the analyst is compelled
> to re-live elements of this infantile history through his counter-
> transference, his internal response to the analysand.
>
> (Bollas 1987: 200)

Searles (1972) comes at this necessity from a different angle, in a
lengthy paper reprinted in *Countertransference and Related Subjects*
(Searles 1979), where part of his argument is that the patient needs
an analyst who will understand them and respond to them in the
right way, just as a baby needs a mother who will understand her
and respond to her correctly. He believes that innate in a human
being's potentialities, from infancy onwards, there is 'an essentially
psychotherapeutic striving' (Searles 1979: 459). As a baby 'teaches'
her mother to become 'a whole and effective mother', so the patient
makes the effort to enable the analyst to become a whole and effective analyst to him or her (p. 459). A simple example that Searles
gives is of a non-obsessive patient teasing the analyst's obsessive
fussing over the lighting in the office, in an attempt to help the
analyst fulfil his emotional potentiality. And, very convincingly, his
longer case examples illustrate how significantly he was 'cured' in
one respect or another by severely disturbed patients. In an example

of this, he relates the story of one patient regretting that her mother did very little for her as a child (and as an adult); but in one session, instead of the usual tension, there was a different quality to the atmosphere. The patient said she felt unusually calm and relaxed and asked Searles if he reacted differently when she felt so. He did, although he did not tell her so – and later regretted he had not told her. She commented that she could imagine her father holding her and cuddling her, but not her mother. It was as if she had created in Searles the calm and the holding that she needed. It is interesting that, in his later discussion of his examples, Searles (1979: 427–30) comments that he believes that acknowledging these therapeutic feelings in the therapist that come from the patient is generally to be recommended.

We can now see why this chapter is headed 'the authentic self'. The struggles of the analyst to understand and work through counter-transference and projective identification can be just as authentic as the more explicit demands of Bugental, May or Rogers for authenticity and genuineness. The effort to get in touch with what is going on at a deep level within oneself is an authentic quest. The reluctance of the analysts to talk about authenticity is perhaps more a question of a way of talking. But to us the authenticity is transparent and obvious.

The second level of empathy

The innate psychotherapeutic striving that Searles describes fits well with Snyder's remark that empathy is developmentally based: 'We are born with the capacity for deep empathic attunement ... our freedom to feel what we feel, and perceive what we perceive, to trust our experience and our intelligence is critically dependent on the empathic attunement of primary caretakers' (Snyder 2000: 109). In Chapter 2, we started to describe three levels of empathy (see Table 2.2). In this chapter, we turn to what might be called Phase 2, 'Column 2 empathy', which is sometimes called 'deep empathy'. Hart (1999) describes this briefly as follows: 'In deep empathy a line is crossed toward a more direct knowing of the other that is enabled by a post-conventional epistemic process. The activity of knowing moves toward subject–object transcendence or a loosening of self/other boundaries' (pp. 115–16). This level does not exclude the first level of empathy described in Chapter 2, but it describes a more refined quality: knowing the client more directly, the capacity to be as it were 'in their shoes', of seeing through their eyes, but at the same time retaining one's own identity. 'The therapist senses what it is like to be where the person is, yet always maintains [his or her] own individuality' (Mahrer *et al.* 1994: 189). This quality of being able to pass to and fro between the client's experience and one's own is mentioned by a number of writers: 'a bold swinging, demanding the most intense stirring of one's being into the life of the other' (Buber 1988: 71); 'imagining what the client is wishing, feeling, and perceiving so vividly and concretely that you experience the existence of the client as your own while remaining in your own existence' (Heard 1995: 251). Hart (1999) observes that the potential always exists 'for distortion and the basic confusion regarding "what is mine and what is theirs" . . . and it is necessary to constantly "check out" material with the client and "check in" with oneself' (pp. 116–17).

It is interesting to see that Hart includes many of the features that this chapter has already discussed and relates these to empathy. He alludes to the therapist experiencing body sensations that appear to come from the client, such as dissociation, or physical feelings of rage. He refers to the need to check countertransferential projections. He refers to projective identification, while acknowledging that the meaning of that term is open to great variation.

Hart wonders whether projective identification, whereby the therapist is 'possessed' (Segal 1964: 14) by parts of the client, is similar to the quality of being 'carried along by' or reacting in unexpected ways such as Carl Rogers describes:

> When I can relax and be close to the transcendental core of me, then I may behave in strange and impulsive ways in the relationship, ways in which I cannot justify rationally, which have nothing to do with my rational thought processes. But these strange behaviors turn out to be right, in some odd way.
>
> (Rogers 1980: 129)

We have noted, as Hart also does, that in Rogers' early writings, there is an 'as if' quality to empathy, but Hart observes that Rogers moves from 'as if' to entering the world of the client 'through an act of alignment'. 'As the therapist enters deeply into the client's world, he or she experiences becoming the other and forming one merged self' (Hart 1999: 119). The self of the therapist becomes the instrument, much as Grotstein (1994) has described, from a psychoanalytic perspective. Using the self in this way paradoxically requires setting aside the self, or in Rogers' (1980: 143) words, 'you lay aside your self'. As Hart (1999: 119) concisely puts it, 'as ego defensiveness decreases, one is free to experience the other more directly and spontaneously'.

This level of empathy is therefore given different names: deep empathy, countertransference, projective identification. Some analysts (e.g. the Jungian Kenneth Lambert) identify empathy with concord- ant countertransference. Tansey and Burke (1989) prefer projective identification as the equivalent: 'when empathy occurs, projective identification is always involved . . . Empathy is the outcome of a radically, mutual interactive process between patient and therapist in which the therapist receives and processes projective identifica- tions from the patient' (p. 195). Kohut (1980a: 450–1) wonders if empathy and intuition are the same, but concludes that empathy is open to rational investigation, whereas intuition is not. It is impor- tant to remember, however, that in all the relationships described above, there is a clear difference between the therapist and the client or patient. It is a kind of meeting, no matter how intimate the meeting may be. It is not until we get into the transpersonal type of relationship, described in Chapter 4, that the idea of meeting gives way to the idea of merging.

Kohut is perhaps the principal exponent of empathy in the psy- choanalytic tradition, empathy being one of the cornerstones of self-psychology practice. The relationship to the therapist in self- psychology takes several forms, including twinship (someone in the world is like me), idealizing (there is someone that I can look up to) and mirroring (someone completely understands me). The therapist attempts to establish and maintain an 'empathic' position, through which the therapist's words and actions remain as close as they can to the patient's inner experience. This is also known as 'mirroring', meeting the need of the patient to find someone who completely understands them. It is this that helps make the therapeutic con- nexion and allows interpretative work to take place. It is not in itself a curative factor, but it provides the necessary context for therapy – in that respect Kohut is, of course, like Rogers listing empathy as one of the core conditions for therapy. [See also the companion volume in the series, *The Therapeutic Environment*, by Hazler and Barwick (2001) for the core conditions.] 'Mirroring creates a reflect- ive relationship that mitigates the patient's aloneness, confirms the truth of the patient's feelings, memories, and conceptual frameworks within a particular context of past experience and distress . . . Kohut saw all effective therapeutic action as taking place in a field of em- pathy' (Hamburg 1991: 348). Through empathic response on the part of the therapist, 'transmuting internalization' helps brings about change, although an essential ingredient that is not found in the humanistic school's emphasis on empathy is that change also comes about through empathic failures, which do not traumatize, but gradually help shift the importance of the therapist as an internal self-object to the patient's more autonomous self. 'It is of note that the implication of this theoretical view is that structural change results from moments of difference, not consistent identity, or therapeutic attunement' (Hamburg 1991: 348). Hamburg suggests that this provides a link to the otherwise very different approach of Lacan, who would see mirroring as freezing 'the therapeutic relationship into an undifferentiated realm of symbiotic illusion' (Hamburg 1991: 349). It is interesting when comparing terms to note that Mearns and Thorne (1988: 56), from the person-centred position, similarly use the image of the mirror in discussing empathic sensitivity, citing Rogers (1986) and an article by a patient of Rogers, who saw him as 'a magical mirror . . . I looked into the mirror to get a glimpse of the reality that I am' (Slack 1985).

Light is thrown upon the process that we are describing, call it empathy or any of the other titles, through the concept of inter-subjectivity and through field theory, where 'patient and therapist together form a psychological system' (Trop and Stolorow 1997: 279). Hart describes this as a form of participant-observation into which the therapist enters in a kind of play; Grotstein (1994) also uses the term 'drama', hence the reference above to Stanislavsky. Winnicott (1971) uses 'play' in a slightly different sense, related to the free play of childhood: 'Psychotherapy is done in the overlap of two play areas, that of the patient and that of the therapist. If the therapist cannot play he is not suitable for the work' (p. 54). And as Hart points out, special metaphors for the therapeutic encounter are found in Winnicott's (1971) 'potential space', Heidegger's (1993) 'clearing', and Buber's (1985) 'between'.

Such phrases share with the intersubjective therapists a focus on the 'between' rather than on either the client or the therapist. Concepts of dialogue and social field become much more important from an intersubjective perspective. There are even some inter-subjective theorists who go so far as to claim that there is no such thing as a separate self, and that all we need is the concept of a field (e.g. Wheway 1997; Sapriel 1998; Wheeler 1998), where the emphasis is all on context and the between. This has happened both in the psychodynamic and in the humanistic-existential traditions. The Jungian tradition has always had a notion of the therapist and the patient being engaged in a common purpose, in equality and mutuality, although this may stress more the importance of 'being together' than what is 'between' them.

Dialogue emerges from the between, based, for example, in one Gestalt tradition, both on experiencing the other person as he or she really is and showing the true self, sharing phenomenological awareness. (We are aware that some Gestalt therapists such as Yontef have no use for the concept of a true self.) Dialogue is what emerges when you and I come together in an authentically contactful manner. Dialogue is not 'you plus I', but rather what emerges from the interaction, which may happen when both parties make themselves present. It can happen only if the outcome is not controlled or determined by either party. Buber is an eloquent and persuasive proponent of dialogic existentialism (Friedman 1976) and has inspired others, notably Yontef, who identifies five characteristics that mark the dialogic relationship: (1) inclusion, (2) presence, (3) commitment to dialogue, (4) no exploitation and (5) that dialogue is lived (Yontef 1993: 221–37). One of the most striking exponents of this view is Hycner, who says that ultimately we have to admit that we are wounded and incomplete and to use that very knowledge in the work. 'The therapist must incessantly struggle to bring his woundedness into play in the therapy . . . In fact, it is this struggling that develops the self of the therapist. This struggling is so central because ultimately the therapist's self is the instrument which will be used in therapy' (Hycner 1993: 15). This is perhaps one of the central insights that we are trying to promulgate in this book.

If Kohut and Rogers from their different positions see empathy as providing the context, Clarkson (1995) makes the point that empathy is arguably part of the reparative relationship in therapy – one of the five elements that she has stressed in helping us to understand the breadth of the therapeutic relationship. She writes: 'For most human beings who have had deficiency experiences in terms of being listened to and understood for most of their childhood (and adult) lives, the therapeutic effect of the provision of these experiences must be due to reparation of some kind' (Clarkson 1995: 88). Countertransference, particularly of the complementary kind, like transference, would appear to describe more a *repetition* of the past in the therapist–client relationship, rather than a *correction* of the past. Clarkson also distinguishes empathy as essentially supportive, which distinguishes an empathic response from an interpretation, the latter often being the type of intervention therapists make when drawing upon transference and countertransference.

It is, as we have already noted, to Rogers that we would be expected to look for the significance of empathy. Mearns and Thorne (1988: 26) include the development of empathy in their chapter on the person-centred counsellor's use of self. They also borrow terms in their chapter on empathy (pp. 39–58) from Gendlin (1981), who made a 'striking contribution to our understanding of the empathic process' (p. 47) – terms such as 'focusing', 'the edge of awareness' and the use of 'handle-words' to try and get an accurate fit on the felt sense in the counsellor of what the client is experiencing, as well as of underlying feelings of which the client is not yet aware. Further explorations of empathy from a person-centred perspective are published in *Rogers' Therapeutic Conditions, Vol. 2: Empathy* (Haugh and Merry 2001).

Hart (1999) observes that, 'in empathic inclusion it is quite natural to experience the unconditional positive regard, even love, that Rogers advocated so strongly' (p. 117). Hart compares this to the awakening of natural compassion (Dass and Gorman 1996) or the opening of the heart chakra described in tantric yogic tradition (Nelson 1994) or the experience of moving from 'I–It' to 'I–Thou' for Buber (1970).

There has been criticism of therapists over-empathizing and of the assumption of therapist correctness by the intersubjectivists, just as Samuels has questioned an over-emphasis on countertransference accuracy. As we comment below, some analysts have warned against the temptation to over-identify with the patient. Britton (1998: 4), also from a psychoanalytic perspective, has drawn attention to the danger of trusting intuition, another important facet of the therapist's use of self, which we discuss below.

Identification

Is empathy a form of identification? The analyst Fliess (1942: 213) clearly states that the analyst's attitude is based on empathy, which, in turn, depends on a 'transient' or 'trial' identification with the patient. Feltham and Dryden (1993) define a trial identification as 'a skill used by the psychodynamic counsellor who seeks to understand his client's inner world by empathic attempts to identify with her and/or with the significant people in her story' (pp. 199–200). Langs (1982) has some similar thoughts. Identification as a concept is closely linked with internalization, which is the subject of another book in this series (Wallis and Poulton 2001).

It is common to conceptualize therapist identification as being on a continuum: the midpoint and its surrounding portion can be regarded as the 'area of optimal identification'. At the right extreme of the continuum is over-identification, where the therapist becomes overly enmeshed in the client's material; on the far left is disidentification, involving a failure to identify with the client effectively (see Watkins 1989: 88). There are some further remarks on the general understanding of identification in Hinshelwood's (1989) excellent text, where he mentions introjective identification, projective identification and adhesive identification.

Friedman (1996) has drawn attention to the way in which Buber has talked about 'inclusion' and 'imagining the real'. By inclusion, Buber means a remarkable swinging over to the side of the other with the most intense activity, so that one experiences concretely what the other person is thinking, feeling and willing. Inclusion

> is the extension of one's own concreteness, fulfilment of the actual situation of life, the complete presence of the reality in which one participates.
>
> (Buber 1985: 97)

> I experience . . . the specific pain of another in such a way that I feel . . . this particular pain as the pain of the other.
>
> (Buber 1988: 60)

Watkins (1978) uses the term 'resonance' and calls it a type of identification. He likens this phenomenon to two pianos put side by side: note A is hit on one of them and the A string in the other piano resonates in sympathy. In the kind of therapy, he says, where this approach is used, what actually happens is that the therapist sets up an ego state (Berne 1961) corresponding to the client and puts energy into that. In that way, the therapist can be with the client from the inside and share the client's subjectivity. Resonance is that inner experience within the therapist during which time he or she co-feels, co-enjoys, co-suffers and co-understands with the client; a type of identification that is temporary, in the here-and-now, an act of conscious choice.

Many different therapeutic schools appear, therefore, to suggest that the therapist needs to open to the unconscious, to allow an interpersonal merger to occur, to foster what Balint (1968) called a 'harmonious, interpenetrating mix-up', to take a receptive stance, and accept the forces from the depths that push the work in new directions. As we have already observed, the possibilities depend largely on the therapist's subjective feeling of readiness to take it on, which includes the capacity to experience her or his own hatred and rage (Sullivan 1989: 133; see also Winnicott 1975: 194–203).

It is also possible to see how over-identification can become a difficulty. Ekstein and Wallerstein (1972: 156) have an example, where a therapist in supervision came up against this problem. In the supervisory hour, the therapist stated that the patient in her appearance and behaviour resembled his own wife and he could only think of the poor devil of a husband. Quite clearly this identification touched off a key problem for him and would have to be dealt with before he could focus on the problems of learning and technique in relation to his work with the patient.

Similarly, Bychowski, in discussing a paper by Searles and others on violence in schizophrenia comments:

> As I go over the cases presented, my principal disagreement is with Dr Searles' by now well-known countertransference interpretations. I must admit that in his former publications I had been struck by his most unusual identification with his psychotic patients. In the present paper he intersperses his excellent interpretations of the patient's dynamics with his 'countertransference' interpretations which, I must confess, seem to me arbitrary and farfetched . . . To read Dr Searles' further exposition of his and supposedly the other therapists' murderous impulses – apparently his entourage is also filled with all sorts of violent feelings toward the patients – is to be subjected to further shocks. One cannot help asking oneself: How can one help a patient if one identifies with him to such an extent, and how can one recognise one's own feelings if one is so ready to distort them by uncritical counteridentification?
>
> (Searles *et al.* 1973: 337–8)

Searles, in reply, stands by his belief that the therapist's own feelings are 'priceless data', which do not have to be assumed to be 'intrusive reactions' from his or her own unexplored childhood (Searles *et al.* 1973: 357–8).

Although this concern comes from the psychoanalytic wing, humanistic therapists are equally suspicious of over-identification. In Gestalt therapy it is called 'confluence', a situation where the necessary boundaries between therapist and client become eroded in a pathological way. 'Confluence is a phantom pursued by people who want to reduce difference so as to moderate the upsetting experience of novelty and otherness' (Polster and Polster 1973: 92). Or, as Zinker (1978) puts it, 'The therapist's greatest enemy is that state in which he finds himself deeply identified with his client, embedded in the other's psychological skin . . . Creative conflict, or simply good contact, is sacrificed for routine interactions which are flat, static and safe' (p. 46). This is reminiscent again of Lacan's criticism of mirroring as symbiotic illusion.

Nevertheless, some forms of confluence may be healthy and valuable. For Freud (1921), identification is something quite primitive, but what we are thinking of here is something sophisticated, which goes beyond the ordinary therapeutic set-up, that is neither what Watkins (1989) calls 'optimal identification' nor over-identification. Liss (1996) writes about 'the identification method' and describes how he uses this both in individual and in group work. Hart gives this example from the work with one client. While the client has excitement for a new project, anytime he seems to get up a head of steam, he 'fogs out', becomes confused, physically weak and appears quite helpless. As the therapist sits with the client, he too becomes 'foggy', dissociated and lost. There is a physical sense of his head clouding as if some dulling, narcotic fog has rolled in. Added to the physical sensation are feelings of helplessness, disappointment and confusion; an image of a tiny baby with his hands clenched on his chest pops up in the therapist's awareness. The therapist has the need to rattle his head back and forth, to slap himself gently to 'snap out of it' so that he can communicate this experience back to the client. Understandably, the client has tremendous difficulty communicating verbally while in this state, but when the therapist describes his own experience, the client says, 'That's it, that's just what it is like' (Hart 2000: 263). Again this has strong similarities with embodied countertransference, and goes a long way to suggesting that empathy, identification and countertransference are often different terms used to describe various types of similar experiences. However, we have to emphasize once more that the therapist remains the therapist, and the other remains the other: we are talking here about meeting not merging, encounter not interbeing.

Intuition and imagination

One of the four basic functions of consciousness identified by Jung is intuition, meaning for Jung a sense of where something is going, of what the possibilities are, without conscious proof or knowledge

(Samuels 1985: 62). Sedgwick (1993) observes that Jung stresses the therapist's use of his intuitive faculty. Feltham and Dryden (1993: 97–8) attribute this psychological function to Jung as well, although they prefer to seek an explanation for it as 'rapid subliminal perception and deduction'. The psychoanalyst Britton (1998: 97–108), in writing his own essay on intuition, quotes Bion: 'an evolution, namely the coming together, by a sudden precipitating intuition, of a mass of apparently unrelated incoherent phenomena which are thereby given coherence and meaning not previously possessed' (Bion 1967: 127). We have noted already that Britton warns against overvaluation of intuition, in much the same way as others warn against the dangers of over-identification. Britton adds another feature of the analyst's mental processes, 'phantasy', which he says is very similar to imagination. Both intuition and phantasy/imagination are surely part of Freud's commendation of 'free-floating attention' and Bion's description of 'reverie' in the therapist? We have also referred to Kohut's distinction between intuition and empathy: he describes intuition as 'the rapid and preconscious gathering of a great number of data and the ability to recognise that they form a meaningful configuration, or the one-step recognition of a complex configuration that has been preconsciously assembled' (Kohut 1980a: 451).

Lomas (1994), who devotes a whole book to the subject, links intuition and the capacity to empathize, where he uses intuition to mean 'direct and immediate insight' where 'we are quite unaware of the steps which led to our knowledge'. Elsewhere, Lomas (1999: 130) also links intuition to countertransference. He sees intuition as a quality that some possess to such an extent that it greatly enhances their work, but that it can be developed in the learning process, being 'an attribute of major significance in the selection and teaching of prospective therapists' (Lomas 1994: 11). Sedgwick (1993: 124) observes in his study of Jung and Searles that a highly developed intuition not only provides access to the therapist's own and the client's unconscious, but also enables the therapist to know *when* to mention or interpret feelings. This is indeed important, since a therapist can have both an intuitive idea that he or she may or may not choose to use at the time, but also can intuitively believe that it is right to share an idea or a feeling which on all other criteria seems as yet not to be appropriate. Lomas has referred to this (in a private communication) as having 'red and green lights' in one's mind that say 'stop' or 'go ahead', and he links useful interpretations to common sense, tact, a sense of timing and intuition (Lomas 1994: 32). He also employs the term 'spontaneity' in this connection (Lomas 1999: 78). A rather different angle on intuition also comes from Searles (1965: 337), when he suggests that unconscious intuition can cause a therapist *not* to notice certain processes in the patient, because it is not yet the time to try and integrate these into the therapeutic relationship. Rowan (1993: 14–17) has suggested that there are six quite distinguishable facets that all go under the heading of intuition, so that it is not a single identifiable function. He says that what we have called the instrumental approach uses role-playing intuition, that the authentic approach uses autonomous intuition and that the transpersonal approach uses surrendered intuition.

Personhood

Having elaborated on many terms that connote different aspects (or perhaps the same aspect?) of the therapist's entering into the experience of the patient, or being willing to be impinged upon by the patient, we might try to come to some kind of conclusion about the way in which the therapist functions at this level: that he or she is able to draw upon their whole self, or their real self. Many schools suggest that therapists can only take clients as far as they have gone themselves, and that if the client is to find their real self, it is essential that therapists have found theirs. Friedenberg (1973) describes this as 'personal awareness, depth of real feeling, and above all that one can use one's full powers, that one has the courage to be and use all one's essence in the praxis of being' (pp. 93–4). We are aware that the notion of a real self has been challenged by social constructivism and post-modernism, an issue that is fully covered in the companion volume on *The Self and Personality Structure* (Brinich and Shelley 2002); we are perhaps using a metaphor, but we would assert in this context that the real or true self is not a concept but an experience. It is, as we suggested at the start of this chapter, equivalent to Winnicott's (1965: 187) notion of the True Self. We must also observe that there is a difference between the experience of the real self, where the therapist is independent of the client – ideally ahead of the client in self-awareness and therefore able to respond better to the client – and the inter-subjective self where the self of the therapist can only be known in therapy through the relationship with the client. These are significant differences between the early expression of gestalt therapy and later expressions such as those to be found in Yontef's (1993) later essays.

Once again we find different expressions for a common idea. Bugental (1978) refers to 'presence' in psychotherapy – the nearest thing in the English language to the German word *Dasein*, which is so important in existentialism. Winnicott (1975) lists features of the psychoanalytic setting, which includes 'the analyst would be there, on time, breathing . . . the analyst is much more reliable than people are in ordinary life' (p. 285). But presence is immensely more than just being there physically:

> It's being totally in the situation . . . Presence is being there in body, in emotions, in relating, in thoughts, in every way . . . Although fundamentally presence is a unitary process or characteristic of a person in a situation, accessibility and expressiveness may be identified as its two chief aspects.
>
> (Bugental 1978: 36–7)

However, Bugental also cautions that it is not easy to attain. Certainly it is not a state that can be once achieved and thereafter maintained. 'Rather it is a goal continually sought, often ignored, and always important to the work of psychotherapy' (Bugental and Sterling 1995: 231). It is important for any form of psychotherapy, but for existential work it is absolutely central. It is not part of the way of talking in psychoanalysis, and indeed many psychoanalysts are quite suspicious of it, as if it were claiming too much; but as we have seen, vast numbers of those in the psychodynamic field actually perform in a way which seems to imply it.

The existentialist therapist Rollo May lays explicit stress upon presence. He draws attention to the way in which Karl Jaspers and Ludwig Binswanger emphasize the importance of presence, and to the way in which Carl Rogers also refers to it quite unmistakably. One of the most important things for any therapist is to be aware of whatever blocks the ability to be fully present. 'The therapist's function is to be there (with all of the connotations of *Dasein*), present in the relationship, while the patient finds and learns to live out his own *Eigenwelt*' (May 1983: 163). Presence is perhaps more than genuineness, the first of the core conditions in person-centred therapy, although Mearns and Thorne (1988) refer to genuineness as part of a therapist's 'way of being', which extends far further than the consulting room, into other relationships as well (see also the eight accounts in Spinelli and Marshall (2001) by different therapists on the influence of their model on their life). Mearns and Thorne see genuineness as one of several names for congruence, including in their other synonyms 'realness' and 'authenticity', although confusingly suggesting that a counsellor can be authentic and yet incongruent. They note that congruence needs to be distinguished from empathy, the former term describing the match 'between the counsellor's underlying feelings and her outward behaviour' (Mearns and Thorne 1988: 76).

This ability to be fully present is the classic existentialist demand. It runs all the way through the gestalt, the psychodramatic, the experiential, the dialogical – all the classic humanistic approaches. It is a type of existentialism that includes the spiritual, although that aspect we reserve for Chapter 4. In the humanistic and existential tradition, there is a strong presumption that the therapist will have developed up the Maslow ladder, to the point that it is the authentic (self-actualized) self of the therapist that will engage with the client.

Existentialist thinkers like R.D. Laing emphasize the presence of the therapist and the co-presence of the client. 'Near the end of his life, Laing often talked about the practice of co-presence. He defined it as the practice of non-intrusive attentiveness, a wholesome concern for each other's life and death' (Feldmar 1997: 350).

Carl Rogers, as we have mentioned, is well known for his insistence that it is the genuine qualities of the therapist that offer the best hope for the client. Virginia Satir is particularly strong on the idea that the full personhood of the therapist is the main ingredient in what makes therapy effective in helping the client in turn to achieve full 'personhood', a term that appears to have been coined by her:

> The whole therapeutic process must be aimed at opening up the healing potential within the patient or the client. Nothing really changes until that healing potential is opened. The way is through the meeting of the deepest self of the therapist with the deepest self of the person, patient or client. When this occurs, it creates a context of vulnerability – of openness to change.
>
> (Satir 1987: 25)

The personhood of the therapist is discussed from a number of angles in the book of that name edited by Brothers (2000). For example, Lander and Nahon describe their work with couples using integrity therapy, where the personhood of the therapist is the very essence of therapy. For them, integrity comprises honesty, responsibility and increased emotional involvement with others. Self-disclosure (see also below) is normal in this approach:

We believe that the traditional prescribed therapists' secretiveness or neutrality denies the human relationship which they aim to foster, thereby limiting their effectiveness. Consequently, we encourage therapists, when they are comfortable to do so, to share their past misdeeds and their present struggles to behave with scrupulous integrity. This atmosphere encourages the development of meaningful human relationships with others which allows for the transcendence of disabling problems.

> (Lander and Nahon 2000: 33)

In the same book, which is a tribute to the work of Satir, Cowley and Adams write an inspiring account of her work, where part of her use of the various facets of herself in therapy includes her imperfections – a point we return to in the next section on the wounded healer:

Virginia claimed the right to be imperfect and still be helpful. Even though trust, authenticity, warmth, respect, and generativity were held up as therapeutic ideals, conscious effort was focused on legitimizing the idea that limitations are also an integral part of any real human being and/or the relationships people co-create together.

> (Cowley and Adams 2000: 54)

If the humanistic schools are more insistent about the presence of the whole person of the therapist, we should not assume that representatives of other schools think otherwise. It is, for example, clear to Jung that the therapist's 'personality' as a whole is the chief instrument at his or her disposal: 'We have learned to place in the foreground the personality of the doctor himself as a curative or harmful factor . . . The crucial thing is no longer the medical diploma, but the human quality'; the psychoanalyst Searles similarly states that countertransference, including the therapist's 'personality and especially his sense of identity [are] of the greatest and most reliable research and therapeutic value' (both cited in Sedgwick 1993: 120).

The wounded healer

If it has been said that the therapist can only take the client as far as he or she as the therapist has gone, this does not mean that therapists have to be perfect – to be perfectly analysed, to have achieved optimum maturity. Many of the most significant writers on human-istic and Jungian psychotherapy concur that the therapist is effect-ive because he or she is closely in touch with their 'shadow' side, as Jungians might put it (Page 1999). Sullivan (1989) has written that it is 'only by facing and accepting our own madness can we hope to help our patients face theirs'. Rogers has said in an interview:

> The therapist needs to recognize very clearly the fact that he or she is an imperfect person with flaws which make him vulner-able. I think it is only as the therapist views himself as imperfect and flawed that he can see himself as helping another person. Some people who call themselves therapists are not healers, because they are too busy defending themselves.
>
> (Baldwin 2000: 36)

A useful summary of the work on this is to be found in Miller and Baldwin (2000), who remark that 'creativity is constantly renewed despite, or perhaps because of, the wounded-healer's vulnerability' (p. 258).

In the Jungian tradition, it is urged that the therapist should be further along the path to individuation than the patient. It is the therapist who has experienced and healed his or her own wounds who offers most hope to the patient. The concept of the wounded healer is very important in this tradition, as Hillman (e.g. 1979) has urged many times, emphasizing the archetypal element in this. Guggenbühl-Craig (1971), a Jungian psychiatrist, explores the image of the wounded healer, showing how easy it is to split the therapist and patient into healthy therapist and ill patient, masking the true situation that the therapist has wounds and that the patient has the capacity to heal himself or herself. The classic paper on this is that by Groesbeck (1975), who shows the intricacy of the conscious and unconscious relationships involved. Samuels (1985: 187–91), in reviewing the Jungian literature, summarizes the idea of an inner healer, saying that a fundamental process in the therapist may be described 'as activation of the inner healer of the patient which performs a healing function for him' (p. 191). At the start of therapy, there is a projection on to the therapist of the inner healer of the patient, which is gradually put back into the patient. The wounds in the therapist 'facilitate empathy with the patient, but the danger is identification' (p. 189).

What is surprising is that psychoanalytic literature is woefully lacking in any reference to the idea of the wounded healer. A search of a massive collection of psychoanalytic articles only reveals a mere handful of references to the idea, and then they are citing Jungian references. Even Searles, one of the most open of analytic writers, somewhat defensively supports his description of troubled emotional responses in the supervisor as being potentially indicative of the reflection (parallel) process: 'My own experience strongly suggests that no therapist ever reaches such a high degree of self-awareness and technical competence as to be consistently free from important involvements of the kind I have been describing' (Searles 1965: 174). It is our impression that in respect of the concept of the wounded healer, while psychoanalysts may acknowledge their fallibility and vulnerability, these are weaknesses that require further therapy and supervision, rather than paths towards deeper healing. Buckley, in a review of the object relations therapist Harry Guntrip's collected papers, is surely right about the example he could offer to the psycho-analytic community when he concludes: 'Guntrip is a vivid example of the "wounded healer" so familiar to anthropologists who have studied the life histories of shamans in other cultures. When he wrote that "real psychotherapy does as much for the therapist as for the patient" (Guntrip 1968: 354), he was revealing a truth not often faced' (Buckley 1997: 582).

Self-disclosure

We finally come to a question which hangs over all that has been described to this point in this chapter: how much does the therapist reveal of her or his inner processes, particularly as related to what is taking place in the here-and-now of the consulting room, but also where it is felt to be relevant, of her or his everyday life as well? The engagement of the therapist that we described in Chapter 2 presumes that little of what we discussed there will be revealed: that is the point of that particular way of using the self – that the self of the therapist is kept hidden so as not to interfere with what the client wants to say, or with what the client is experiencing. Of the many ways in which the therapist more actively uses the self that we have covered in this chapter, it is obvious that empathic interventions only become empathic when they are openly shared. It would probably be agreed by every therapeutic approach that other aspects of the therapist's thought processes – identification, intuition, imagination – will also be shared when it seems appropriate, and made relevant to the client without necessarily revealing anything about the therapist: 'I can imagine how you might be feeling...if I were in your position, I might consider...etc.' But there is much less agreement across orientations as to whether the therapist might say: 'Just at this moment I'm feeling (such and such) in myself', or 'I remember when I went through a similar experience'.

First impressions also suggest that if we are going to look for any disclosure by the therapist that is at all personal, it is to the humanistic and existential therapies that we might expect to find support and examples. On the whole, the psychoanalytic tradition opposes self-disclosure as interfering with the transference, although we shall show that it is not quite so clear-cut as that. The more cognitive and behavioural approaches seem to find little point in self-disclosing or temptation to do so, except perhaps in giving feedback about how the client seems to the therapist – hardly self-disclosure. Intersubjectivists share with their clients their own conflicts of how much of their feelings to reveal. Hycner, for example, mentions an instance when:

> sensing her greater openness I took a major risk and I told her how I had often felt like a phantom to her. The potential for meeting outweighed the risks of 'mismeeting'. In fact, I believed that it was *essential* for her to deal with this issue, since most likely she was dealing with other people in a similar manner. Though my comment hurt her feelings initially, it became a turning point in the therapy.
>
> (Hycner 1993: 72)

It is also in the humanistic and existential tradition that we find full discussions of different types and levels of self-disclosure. One of the most basic aspects of this is drawn out by an exchange of views between Carl Rogers and Rollo May. Rogers is well known for his insistence on genuineness and congruence in the therapist, but in practice (for example, as shown in the book edited by Farber *et al.* 1996) he appears never to have expressed any negative feelings. May criticizes this:

> Rogers has, of course, been in the forefront of those insisting on respect for the patient. But is not respect best and most profoundly shown by openly admitting anger, hostility and conflict with another, but at the same time not withdrawing one whit from the relationship? Indeed, such 'inclusion of the

negative' normally can make a relationship, and the mutual respect in it, more solid and trustworthy.

(May 1980: 216)

Once this is stated, it appears rather obvious that a therapist who believes that genuineness is important (and humanistic practitioners typically do) must be willing to express negative emotions whenever this could be therapeutic. This will often involve self-disclosure.

Shadley (2000) has laid out a useful range of types of self-disclosure, derived from her research:

- *Intimate interaction*. The therapist tends to open up through verbal and non-verbal expressions of therapeutic responses, often with references to present or past personal issues. Sometimes this is inevitable, as for example when the therapist gets pregnant. But some therapists, perhaps more women than men, rely on it a great deal.
- *Reactive response*. The expression of verbal or non-verbal responses revealing emotional connectedness within the therapeutic relationship, without revealing personal experiences of the therapist's outside life. For example, the therapist may cry at something the client has said. Hill (1989) found that this kind of self-disclosure is particularly valuable in relation to outcome. It goes well with an 'I–Thou' type of emotional connection and immediacy.
- *Controlled response*. The therapist maintains a slight distance by limiting self-disclosures to past experiences, anecdotes, non-verbalized feelings or literary parallels. The therapist chooses carefully which stories or other elements will be most valuable.
- *Reflective feedback*. The therapist offers impressions of client issues, or asks questions that reveal a point of view, but seldom shares personal information or strong emotional reactions. This is perhaps the standard behaviour taught on courses.

These are stances that the therapist may cultivate more or less consciously. But it has to be said that this set of choices is quite uncharted territory for most therapists of all persuasions. A huge effort of education is needed to let therapists know that all these possibilities are used in the field. An unpublished study of self-disclosure concludes:

The data indicates [*sic*] that whilst therapists *do* choose when and how to self-disclose, the reasons for doing so *are* carefully and cautiously considered. Additionally, although disclosing information to the client *does* betray the assumptions relating to their training and theoretical approach, the rationale is congruent with *how* they view the fundamental working philosophy of emphasising the 'person-to-person' relationship.

(King 2000: 36, emphasis in original)

Within psychodynamic traditions, the Jungian position offers a wide range of interest in self-disclosure, with those at the more Kleinian (psychoanalytic) end of the spectrum probably being the least likely to say much about themselves. Sedgwick comments that, for Jung (and Searles, with whom he compares him), therapeutic anonymity is almost as unnecessary as the pretension to neutrality. If the therapist experiences affects, and uses himself or herself in the work with the client, this implies that there will be some expression of this. Jung believes in spontaneity (Sedgwick 1993: 123). There would be little point in the analyst discovering the archetype of the wounded healer if he or she never shared this knowledge with the patient. 'If the analyst has been moved by his patient, then the patient is more aware of the analyst as a healing presence. This frees the patient to have communication with his inner healer, identified as his potential' (Samuels 1985: 189). Another Jungian writes:

> I don't conceal myself. I frequently use myself as therapeutic instrument, and I don't try to be anonymous. Often I share my feelings with analysands – if the feelings are relevant . . . I think an analysand is entitled to reactivity from his analyst. Of course, I may temper my reactions. It may be that the ego of the person I am working with is fragile, and if I get angry, for instance, I will hold back. But I would surely sooner or later be able to say, 'You know, ten minutes ago I was terribly angry at you, and the reason was . . .'. But if the patient is not too fragile, I might say, 'The hell you say, you goddamn fool'. Or I might laugh, or cry – any of these reactions is possible.
>
> (Wheelwright 1982: 117)

Family therapy, which often involves live supervision, may well mean obvious self-disclosure of therapist's feelings and thoughts to the family group. Indeed, in group therapy, even of the psychoanalytic sort, the therapist is more transparent. However, there is a major difference between, on the one hand, the model of Foulkes and Anthony (1965: 62) and the Institute of Group Analysis where greater openness by the therapist, owning personal feelings, acts as a model for the group members as to how to relate; and, on the other hand, the model of Bion (1961, 1962) and the Tavistock Institute of Human Relations, which tends towards a somewhat distant and esoteric group consultant, who makes group interpretations and is more concerned with the actual group than the relationships of the individual members to one another within it, except inasmuch as they are indicative of basic assumptions in the group. Here self-disclosure is almost non-existent, although of course Bion (1961: 29–40), in his early experiences in groups, was ready to disclose that he did not know what was happening, and was hammered for it!

The humanistic tendency is to self-disclose, with a humanistic psychologist, Jourard, writing the classic work on self-disclosure as a general form of interaction. Jourard (1968, 1971) found in his research that self-disclosure is the optimum way of building up a human relationship of the 'I Thou' kind. For the person-centred therapist, congruence is one of the main core conditions, which is likely to involve self-disclosure to be fully responsive to the client. Perhaps one of the most extreme examples of this in the British literature is the person-centred therapist Thorne's naked embrace with a particular client (Thorne 1987), where he claims this event was both at a stage of 'deep mutuality' and was a 'direct response to her overwhelming fear of fragmentation and of corruption' (Dryden 1993: 115). Elsewhere this is held up as a 'striking example' of congruence (Mearns and Thorne 1988: 88). It is an instance of self-disclosure or self-exposure indeed, which extends to the physical. But we also have to recall the even more bold experiments in the 1960s, following the existentialist psychoanalyst R.D. Laing's innovative ideas in the Kingsley Hall community in London (e.g. Barnes and Berke 1973). Questions of such extreme self-exposure raise questions about boundaries, but similar questions about boundaries exist in milder instances of self-disclosure too, where therapists of different orientations have the same regard for the importance of boundaries, but interpret the precise point of them differently. Spinelli (2001) quotes the example of one therapist, who had great success with a difficult patient using a treatment that included talking about his childhood, his marriages, his despair with certain patients, the youth culture, TV and movies, extending sessions, going on walks together, inviting her to his home, providing her with meals, and so on. This seems quite a radical take on boundaries, but Spinelli appears to be quite taken with it and certainly regards it as legitimate.

Similar issues are raised by Gale (1999). Smith *et al.* (1998) is a useful text on these questions. They discuss the whole question of boundaries in some detail, with a good deal of research evidence. It is particularly oriented towards the question of touch, but its findings are highly relevant to other boundary questions as well.

The core condition of congruence in the person-centred tradition seems to imply self-disclosure, although Mearns and Thorne (1988: 81–2) make it clear that congruence is not the same as self-disclosure: they mean by the latter term other elements of the therapist's life. Congruence refers to the therapist's experience of and with the client, and yet even these feelings are only shared when they are relevant to the immediate concern of the client, are persistent and particularly striking (Mearns and Thorne 1988: 82). While masking dislike of a client is called an incongruent response, it is not clear exactly how a therapist would share this aspect congruently. For comparison, we note the example of the analyst Winnicott, faced with a similar situation, who waited until it was safe to share such a feeling. A patient of his was 'almost loathsome to me for some years'. He recounts that 'it was indeed a wonderful day for me (much later on) when I could actually tell the patient that I and his friends had felt repelled by him, but that he had been too ill for us to let him know. This was also an important day for him, a tremendous advance in his adjustment to reality' (Winnicott 1975: 196). But, again from within the analytic orientation, Searles (1965: 26) writes: 'I have become much freer to express and make therapeutic use of previously suppressed scornful feelings toward patients, finding that these do not destroy, but rather help to activate the therapeutic relatedness'. Lomas (1999) is the most obvious proponent of therapist honesty in British psychodynamic writing, who, while recommending that it is unwise to 'indulge thoughtlessly in self-revelations' (p. 65), provides countless examples in his books of speaking his mind, answering patients' questions, and sharing his own dilemmas (see also Lomas 1973, 1994).

When we come to examine psychoanalytic writing more closely, we find quite a number of indications that self-disclosure, of various kinds, is not as unusual as might initially be thought. Freud addressed the issue of self-disclosure as he worked out the most useful techniques to use, but cited various problems that are likely to arise if the therapist responded to the natural wish of the patient that the analyst should say more about him or herself. He concludes that 'experience does not speak in favour of [a] . . . technique of this kind' (Freud 1912a: 118). Yet if we read some of his case histories, and reports of those in analysis with him, it is obvious that he spoke of himself and his family.

Against this, again in the early years of the development of psychoanalysis, we have noted already in Chapter 2 how Ferenczi proposed mutual analysis, and we also referred to the example of Anna Freud as just one of many analysts who clearly have not hidden behind a blank screen. As Greenberg (1995) writes: 'On the one hand we have the testimony of the founder himself that self-disclosure demonstrably undermines our attempts to conduct an analysis. On the other hand we have the testimony of the man who was widely acknowledged to be the foremost clinician of his day that refusing to reveal ourselves demonstrably undermines our attempts to conduct an analysis' (p. 195). He adds that 'the same arguments that Freud and Ferenczi made, putatively based on the same empirical observations, are regularly repeated in contemporary discussions of the issue' (p. 195).

There is a strand of thinking in psychoanalysis that suggests that, just as fostering of the transference will be jeopardized by self-disclosure by the analyst, so towards the end of therapy self-disclosure, or more participation through what is sometimes known as 'real relationship', will help to weaken or dissolve the transference, in preparation for the end of the relationship. Similarly, as Kramer observes, in four times weekly analysis where an intense transference is encouraged, self-revelation is minimal, whereas in once-weekly therapy, where a dependent, regressive transference is not desirable, 'judicious revelation of personal material minimizes' the risk of such extremes (Kramer 2000: 75–6). This appears somewhat manipulative on the part of the therapist and suggests that, indeed, the therapist has the power to regulate the client's feelings. Experience suggests otherwise: transference can be intense, even when there is self-disclosure. Sharing a personal difficulty to try to temper a patient's idealization can lead to even greater idealization, because such honesty can make the therapist into an even more admired figure.

Nuttall (2000: 28–9) argues that this shift in relating takes place in Kleinian psychotherapy, too, so that although it may start in a one-sided way, with the transferential relationship pre-eminent, as therapeutic change occurs the relationship becomes much more person-to-person. Nuttall makes it clear that this cannot be contrived, and adds: 'Physical contact, self-disclosure and social conversation are anathema to a Kleinian therapist' (p. 29). However, Hill describes very different experiences with three Kleinian therapists, only one of whom fits the stereotypical picture of a tightly boundaried analyst. The effect on him 'was not only personally therapeutic in itself but I became aware of my own analytic work both improving and becoming more enjoyable with the whole of myself becoming engaged in a more interesting exploration' (Hill 1993: 469). This is another good example of what moving to the authentic position is like.

An interesting position is set out by Greenberg (1995), who suspects the wrong question is being raised, when it is asked whether analysts should self-disclose. Ferenczi said that it is inevitable that personal information will be revealed. So, first, 'asking a particular question (instead of another that could have been asked); making a particular interpretation; decorating one's office in a particular way; greeting (or not greeting) the patient; wearing a certain kind of tie; cutting one's hair' (Greenberg 1995: 195), and indeed everything that a therapist does or does not do reveals something of the therapist to the perceptive patient. Indeed, Singer (1977: 183) writes: 'what analysts so fondly think of as interpretations are neither exclusively nor even primarily comments about their clients' deeper motivations, but first and foremost self-revealing remarks'. Secondly, everything the therapist does also conceals something: 'Even in moments when we are telling our patients about ourselves we are, consciously or unconsciously, deciding what not to say' (Greenberg 1995: 196). Thirdly, 'whatever is revealed is simply one person's understanding at a given moment – never (despite the patient's and sometimes also the analyst's hopes) the last word on the subject' (Greenberg 1995: 197). Greenberg therefore concludes that:

> it is not particularly useful to attempt to come up with any sweeping statement about self-disclosure. I do not see any advantage to covering a wide range of situations with a one-size-fits-all technical prescription. Rather, our task requires coming to grips with an endless flow of decisions, each made by a particular analyst, with a particular patient, in the context of a particular moment in their relationship. In general, talking about how we arrive at decisions strikes me as more interesting than the particular conclusions we reach, especially when those conclusions are idealized as the only ones that are acceptable.
>
> (Greenberg 1995: 197)

This does seem like the kind of wisdom we should like to urge in this chapter, because it illustrates the openness so characteristic of the authentic self.

Burke and Tansey are more circumspect: 'Although we have attempted to provide clinical guidelines for establishing a "judicious balance" (Tansey and Burke 1989: 3–150), disclosure is an area of technique that remains necessarily ambiguous and uncertain' (Burke and Tansey 1991: 379). Renik, writing in 1995, observes that:

> the whole trend of the past ten years or so toward a theory of technique based on an intersubjective conception of the analytic situation has begun to treat analytic anonymity as a myth and to address the idealizations promoted by the myth . . . the assumption that an analyst can be anonymous and can function as privileged interpreter of a patient's experience ('realistic' versus 'distorted by transference') is rejected. Instead, the patient is recognized to be as much a legitimate interpreter of the analyst's experience as vice versa.
>
> (Renik 1995: 480)

He cites Aron as illustrating the clinical implication of this view:

> I often ask patients to describe anything that they have observed or noticed about me that may shed light on aspects of our relationship . . . I find that it is critical for me to ask the question with the genuine belief that I may find out something about myself that I did not previously recognize . . . in particular, I focus on what patients have noticed about my internal conflicts.
>
> (Aron 1991: 37)

Freud and many of his followers may have rejected Ferenczi, but 'mutual analysis' appears to have survived!

Renik is clear where he stands. After quoting Hoffman's (1994: 198) candid admission that 'the magical aspect of the analyst's authority is enhanced by his or her . . . anonymity. There is a kind of mystique about the analyst that I doubt we want to dispel completely', Renik (1995) adds: 'We may not want to dispel it, but I think we should!' (p. 481). The wish to dispel mystique is the typical authentic aim, and very characteristic of those therapists we have featured in this chapter.

Conclusion

We have covered much in this chapter, which in our opinion is concerned with the central aspect of the therapist's use of self, particularly in long-term therapy. We are not ourselves content to limit the therapist's use of self to those matters discussed in Chapter 2, and we recognize that the material which we go on to discuss in Chapter 4 does not suit every client, even it is part of the understanding of a number of therapeutic orientations. The transpersonal does not have the universal application that we believe the concepts have that are included here. Questions remain, as indeed do disagreements, some of which we have outlined, about exactly how to use the various aspects of the self which the literature identifies, although we have seen more parallels, hidden or distorted sometimes by language, about unmasking the therapist, than we might have imagined before undertaking our search.

There is also the question of how far therapists can learn to use themselves in this way, or whether we are describing qualities which, if not innate (because therapists clearly differ among themselves in their capacity to be empathic, intuitive, etc.), may be personal characteristics that training can enhance or even generate. What are the implications of these uses of the self for training and supervision? That question we address in Chapter 5; but before that we need to examine the third level of the therapist's use of self – the transpersonal self.

CHAPTER 4

The transpersonal self

Beyond the personal

More rarely, but on an increasing scale, theorists are talking about the higher self, the transpersonal self, the Subtle self, the soul, and so forth. The idea often is that certain boundaries are quite different at this level, and may even disappear altogether.

We suggest that much of the therapeutic process is done at the level of ordinary thinking, with the therapist using skills and knowledge and a certain degree of self-perception, as we saw in Chapter 2; and that a smaller amount of therapy – but still a substantial amount – takes place at the level of authentic consciousness, as we saw in Chapter 3. A smaller amount again of therapy is done at the level of a more subtle form of consciousness, which we examine in this chapter.

This subtle consciousness takes the form of an awareness, which we might describe as being similar to what the mystics have described of their own experience. Such a statement might immediately be off-putting to all but those who value the transpersonal contribution to psychotherapy and psychology, although it is important to observe that even supposedly conservative psychoanalysis has in more recent times had its share of authors engaging with dimensions beyond the personal (e.g. Bion 1965; Milner 1987; Eigen 1998; see also Jacobs 2000a). We are describing people who are open to experiences beyond or deep within themselves, who do not simply reproduce the opinions of books, follow societal norms or religious rituals, or conform to what they imagine other people think. This subtle consciousness cannot be 'willed' into existence, but often comes in brief moments, particularly at first when we are new to the experience. It is synonymous with that form of mystical experience that relies a great deal on symbols and images. Subtle awareness is full (depending upon the terms used by different models) of archetypes, of nature spirits, of deity figures, and so forth, all regarded as numinous representations of the divine, or of ultimate reality. There is another expression of mystical experience, which questionably could be described as more advanced, although at this level of thinking we do not favour any notion of a hierarchy any more than we have done elsewhere in this book, as if one sort of experience is 'better' than another. In that other form, all symbols and images are discarded (see Jacobs 2000a: ch. 6). Clearly, such an experience is difficult to describe, since words are essentially symbols themselves. We shall nevertheless attempt to show the relevance of this, too, later in this chapter.

One of the essential features of this form of subtle consciousness is that one's whole sense of boundaries is radically revised. At all the earlier stages, we take it for granted that we end at our skins. What is inside my skin is me, what is outside my skin is not me. This is not only common sense; it is existentialist philosophy. But at the Subtle stage, this does not hold. At a surface level, we are certainly separate; but at a deeper level, we are one. One analogy that has been used is that we are like islands that were originally hills overlooking a plain; the sea rose, the plain sank, and the newly formed islands started to become more and more different and distinct. But they are still part of the same land.

In the psychodynamic field, Bion was one of the first to take this view, and his concept of 'O' is an important feature of his model of therapy. He defines this concept in this way: 'I shall use the sign O to denote that which is ultimate reality represented by terms such as ultimate reality, absolute truth, godhead, the infinite, the thing-in-itself' (Bion 1970: 26). He says that in psychoanalysis both parties can begin to enter into a field that represents ultimate reality. You cannot *know* ultimate reality, you have to *become* it: 'The pathway by which such an experience becomes possible is through the close relationship with another. Psychoanalysis is the investigation of such a relationship and it attempts to open both partners to the mystical experience' (Symington and Symington 1996: 178). In this experience, the normal boundaries disappear, and intuition takes the place of reasoning: psychic reality can only be known through intuition. 'This means that the mental-emotional reality is apprehended directly and not via the senses, Bion's proposition is that the senses block intuition of the psychic reality' (Symington and Symington 1996: 167). In other words, we apprehend the numinous through the relationship with another person – a relationship in which both I and the other are transformed.

More recently, writers like Field, Epstein and others have taken up the view that, at the transpersonal level, boundaries can disappear completely and with therapeutic advantage. Field writes, in the context of issues about projective identification: 'But we are faced with the whole problem of transmission only because we assume that the parties involved are separate entities to begin with. But if, at some unconscious level, *they are already merged* no transfer is required, since in a state of merger what happens to one happens to the other' (Field 1996: 42, emphasis in original). He goes on to speak of the 'four-dimensional state' in which therapist and client can both participate. 'One of the ways in which the four-dimensional state can be experienced is the simultaneous union and separation of self and other. I have in mind those moments where two people feel profoundly united with one another yet each retains a singularly enriched sense of themselves. We are not lost in the other, as in fusion, but found' (Field 1996: 71). Field speaks movingly of the way in which such an experience has a healing power: 'A totally new Gestalt has come into being where separateness and togetherness are simultaneously experienced in all their depth and richness' (p. 73). He is very clear about the feeling of danger that may come to the untried therapist in these circumstances. Our whole culture is dedicated to the proposition that we are responsible for ourselves, and therapy is full of warnings about the dangers of rescuing. But sometimes we have to take these risks.

> Even if you throw a rope to a drowning man, it's no help if he can't take hold of it. In certain situations it may be necessary to jump overboard and go to where he happens to be, even though the therapist takes the risk of drowning too. In practice this means that, when a patient is in such a panic he or she cannot even listen, it may be necessary to abandon the defences that separate the therapist and patient, to go down into the patient's desperation, and consciously share it.
>
> (Field 1996: 98)

Field does not call upon the notion of the collective unconscious, but what he is saying is highly suggestive of that way of thinking, which is so compatible with subtle consciousness, as we indicate below in looking at what Jungians have to say about these matters.

Epstein (1996) suggests that the way into this realm is through meditation. Meditation can, however, bypass this Subtle realm (of symbols and images, archetypes and archetypal dreams, deity figures, and of the heart) as part of seeking a rather different experience, which Wilber (2000) calls the Causal realm (the deep water of spirituality, where all the symbols disappear, and a person is alone with the infinite divine). In therapy this is a real drawback. Without denying the place of meditation, many people find that workshops and rituals offer a more reliable means into the Subtle realm. There are exercises specifically designed to take people into it, though these are best carried out in a group setting with an experienced leader who can guide the process. It may seem that there is a paradox about finding paths into what is essentially a pathless realm, but for those who regard the Subtle realm as just another state of consciousness, quite accessible to everyone, it is no more extraordinary than to say that one can be trained to read an X-ray photograph, or trained to taste wines more expertly. We return to the issue of training in Chapter 5.

The person-centred perspective

In the humanistic and existential tradition, Mearns, Rowan, Mahrer and others have urged that we need to pay attention to the way in which the relationship can actually disappear for brief periods, as the two parties merge into the same identity. Mearns, a person-centred therapist, describes working at relational depth with clients: He asks: 'Is it relational depth which is the special issue, or should we be turning the coin over and asking serious theoretical questions on why this phenomenon is so rare? Is it, for example, because we are too afraid of others or perhaps of our Selves, or both, to risk meeting each other at relational depth?' (Mearns 1996: 306). He then describes what he means by relational depth and gives these examples of clients' description of the therapeutic experience:

It felt as though he was right there, in the garden, with me – like he could see it as well.

It felt as though she was right *inside me* – feeling *me* in the same moment that I was feeling myself.

I knew he felt my terror. But it wasn't just that – it was one of those *I knew he knew I knew* things – like we were communicating at a lot of different levels at the same time.

He also provides examples of what therapists say about such experience, for example:

I had not been *in* that far with a client before . . . I think it happened by accident really . . . I felt so relaxed and at ease with myself. Instead of thinking one step ahead, I just found myself responding to him in the moment – sometimes in ways which were unusual for me. It was amazing how powerful, yet simple, the process was.

Mearns (1996: 307) makes the point that working at relational depth does not imply that this type of experience is occurring all the time. 'The interaction between therapist and client will move around the contact spectrum, at times engaging very deeply and on other occasions much more superficially' (p. 308). He says elsewhere that the idea of *presence* is very important for the whole process:

. . . the counsellor is able to be truly *still* within herself, allowing her person fully to resonate with the client's experiencing. In a sense, the counsellor has allowed her person to step right into the client's experiencing without needing to do anything to establish her separateness. This second circumstance is made much easier for the counsellor if she is not self-conscious.

(Mearns 1994: 8)

This quality has of course been remarked upon many times. For example, Laing, Bion, Hillman and many others have talked about presence in this sort of way. 'Perhaps we might add a little to the theory by suggesting that a prerequisite to achieving this personal "stillness" in relationship with the client is not merely "unselfconsciousness", but also that the therapist is not *afraid*' (Mearns 1996: 309). If this can happen, then 'the therapist who is willing to work with the client at relational depth tries to leave aside conventional ways of responding and projects himself or herself fully into the client's experiencing' (p. 310). This is not easy to do or even (for some therapists) to imagine, because it is not a skill; neither is it a technique that can be learned. Indeed, this ability comes perhaps through *unlearning* some of the injunctions that have been conditioned into therapists in their training and supervision. Therapists who work at this level know when they need to put aside conventional responses, and enter into the unknown, while at the same time fully appreciating the need to hold the usual boundaries, albeit for the time being themselves held back from immediate consciousness. It is possible for therapists to function on a number of different levels at once.

The humanistic-existential perspective

Mahrer, a leading theorist and practitioner in the humanistic-existential tradition, describes this type of involvement as 'experiential listening', a kind of listening that involves a complete sharing of the client's phenomenal world:

> Experiential therapy rests on the assumption that altered states are available wherein the therapist and patient can integrate with one another. The personhood and identity of one can assimilate or fuse with that of the other. The therapist can become a part of the personality of the patient.
>
> (Mahrer 1983: 138)

The therapist and client can integrate with one another. The personhood and identity of one can assimilate or fuse with that of the other, and then the therapist enters the same experience that is currently occurring in the client. Mahrer teaches workshops on this subject and has produced a short manual (Mahrer 1989) on the actual procedures involved, as well as a much fuller account, which goes into more detail (Mahrer 1996). In this kind of alignment, Mahrer (1993) suggests that 'the therapist literally enters completely into being the person . . . Instead of being empathic with the person, you are fully being the person. Instead of knowing the person's world, you are living it' (pp. 33–4). The therapist suspends the separateness of the self and crosses the threshold of subject–object dichotomy. Mahrer's method is one in which both therapist and client attend not to each other, but to a third centre of attention, the client's problem or life situation: 'The therapist [allows] what the patient is saying to come in and through the therapist' (Mahrer *et al.* 1994: 193).

In a similar technique, Sprinkle (1985) 'mentally views the client and [him]self as one personality' (p. 207). 'When I mentally pictured myself as the client to focus on his or her concerns, I learned that various thoughts and images came into my awareness' (p. 206). The therapist describes what he or she senses, feels and thinks through the client's viewpoint.

Mahrer suggests other ways in which this greater openness to experience can be encouraged. For example, to understand the client's experience, it may be possible for the therapist to reproduce in her or his body whatever the client is describing as going on in his or her own body. The therapist gets into the same position as the client, and if the client says there is a pain in the middle of the back, the therapist 'creates' a pain in the middle of her or his back too. This active approach to empathy can be taught and used, so that the therapist exaggerates what the client is saying, so as to get deeper into the experience and to encourage the client to get deeper into the experience.

It is important to note that deep empathy is not a particular technique, but an activity of more direct knowing that involves a shift in being or consciousness. One technique or another may be helpful only to the extent that they engender such a shift. These authors are describing a type of transpersonal experience that a therapist learns to be open to, not yet another technique that can be introduced at the right moment into a session. Mahrer has related some of the connections he sees with other work: 'Something happens that is different from when the two are face-to-face. I call it "being aligned" ' (Mahrer 1996: 153). It is similar to the phenomenon of linking, which we refer to below. Mahrer indicates how widely held this view is:

> Others talk about the two persons in the therapeutic relation-ship being joined or conjoined, or the therapist being plugged into, merged, or fused with the patient (Binswanger 1958a, 1958b; Fromm, Suzuki and DiMartino 1960; Laing 1962, 1982; Maupin 1965). The distinction between what can occur in a face-to-face relationship and what can occur in the two being closely aligned may well underlie Maslow's (1968) distinction between D and B intimacy-love, Fromm's (1956) distinction between mature intimacy-love and symbolic union, Seguin's (1965) dual or shared intimacy-love, Lewis's (1960) gift or need intimacy, and Binswanger's (1958b) distinction between com-munication and communion.
>
> (Mahrer 1996: 153)

This is an impressive roll call, particularly when one thinks how different some of these writers are.

Buber's (1970, 1985) existentialism, as we saw in the last chapter, is mostly to do with being authentic, but one of the more recent existential writers, van Deurzen-Smith, presents this striking statement:

> Beyond these two dimensions of interpersonal relationships a third level can be recognized. It is the level of the I–Me relationship, or the perfect merging of two beings who totally identify with each other and who operate in absolute self-forgetfulness, aiming at something that transcends their separateness and thus binds them together . . . To a certain degree the existential counselling relationship aims at the mode of the unifying I–Me relationship.
>
> (van Deurzen-Smith 1988: 208–9)

This is a powerful recognition that the distancing of therapist from client is not always useful. It suggests very strongly that it is possible to go beyond empathy into what we are calling linking (see below). Van Deurzen-Smith is not saying, of course, that this is the major part of therapy, or that it is a new form of therapy; she is just trying to name something that many therapists (and others outside the therapy profession) have met with in some form at some time. In saying that it is similar to the relationship that we have with ourselves, she is saying something important.

Similarly, Bugental, who bridges in a unique way the gap between the existential and the humanistic, draws attention to research by Sterling in which the supervisee role-plays the client and the supervisor role-plays the supervisee. Sometimes a curious experience occurs:

> Unexpectedly and suddenly, I lose the ability to maintain the immersion I have been experiencing. The distinctions between 'me' and 'the role-played client' dissolve. It is as though there is a collapse of the separated consciousnesses into one *melded* experience . . . I can't tell which of us is the source of the content I am expressing!
>
> (Sterling and Bugental 1993: 42)

Bugental speculates that if our deepest nature is manifested by the 'meld', we may arrive at a rather different picture of our own nature. He takes this idea further into some transpersonal thoughts.

The Jungian perspective

In the Jungian and psychosynthesis traditions, this is quite familiar territory, and a good deal of material supports this. For example, the Jungian Schwartz-Salant (1984) has spoken in his own terms of this phenomenon, having to do with what he calls the 'subtle body': 'a realm that is felt to be outside normal time sense and in a space felt to have substance. This space, long known as the subtle body, exists because of imagination, yet it also has autonomy' (pp. 10–11). He also uses the term *conjunctio*, taken from alchemy (and from Jung), meaning a joining, such that two become one. Elsewhere he speaks even more deeply of this experience, in discussing a particularly difficult client:

> The process is difficult to describe because it exists within an imaginal reality in which one's attention flows through the heart and out toward another person. In the process imaginal sight emerges, a quality of consciousness that perceives the presence of the archetypal level. This sight can be experienced through the eyes, the body or the emotions, but it is a level of perception that gently penetrates in ways that a discursive process fails to achieve. To the abandoned soul, knowledge without heart feels like abandonment. The heart offers a way to connect without violating the soul.
>
> (Schwartz-Salant 1991: 211)

Samuels (1989) indicates that this all takes place in the imaginal world. This imaginal world is an in-between state, where images take the place of language (Corbin 1969, Hillman 1975). It is between the conscious and the unconscious, and also between the therapist and the client. Both persons have access to it and can share it. It is the therapist's body, the therapist's imagery, the therapist's feelings or fantasies; but these things also belong to the client, and have been squeezed into being and given substance by the therapeutic relationship. Samuels emphasizes that these are *visionary* states, concluding that such experiences may usefully be regarded as religious or mystical. Given the Jungian concept of the collective unconscious, it is perhaps not surprising to find this recognition of the way in which therapist and client are 'joined' at a deeper level.

Indeed, this stratum of the unconscious may be even more extensive, according to some ideas from the perspective of Moreno and psychodrama, where we find a similar concept to the collective unconscious, albeit using a different term, that of 'tele': 'tele could be defined as "the between distance", all of the energies flowing in the distance between two or more . . . Tele as an inter-phenomenon relates to individuals, dyads, groups and the cosmos' (Moreno *et al.* 2000: 72). This emphasis on the 'between' leads to the claim: 'We are relationship therapists. Relationships include relations with people who may be absent or present, animals, objects, values, the deceased, or possibly God' (Moreno *et al.* 2000: 74). And Adam Blatner tells us (Blatner 1994: 296) that tele involves an opening of one's heart and an expanding of one's perspective.

The third level of empathy

In Chapter 2, Table 2.2 describes three levels of empathy. We may ask whether what we have described in this chapter is a deeper form of that empathy which is so vital to every level of the therapeutic process. Hart (1997) has written about transcendental empathy, referring both to transcendental countertransference and to psychological resonance. Liss (1996) refers to 'the identification method' and describes very clearly how he uses this both in individual and in group work. To use it in groups obviously extends the experience still further.

For some therapists, deep empathic experience does not involve a state of fusion but a refined sympathetic resonance (see, for example, Sprinkle 1985; Rowan 1986; Larson 1987). The phenomenon of sympathetic acoustical resonance parallels empathic resonance. When two violins are located in the same room and a string is plucked on one, the string tuned to the same frequency on the other will also vibrate. In a similar phenomenon, therapists may find themselves particularly sensitive to certain information in the other, such as specific emotions, and quickly resonate with and recognize these sensations in the client. Some therapists may be sensitive to feelings in general, others to a wide range of experiences (e.g. thoughts, perceptual style, etc.). Others become skilful in tuning into relevant material in a variety of forms. This is not merely imagining, extrapolating or interpreting cues; the epistemic process is more direct. Subjectivity is suspended to attune with the other.

Gestalt therapy recognizes this as using the self as a 'resonance chamber' (Polster and Polster 1973: 18). Unlike the transient fusion in the experience of alignment (see Mahrer above), the phenomenology of attunement describes the experience of two selves connecting at a particular 'frequency' of experience. Such models as field theory (e.g. Sheldrake 1988; Smith and Smith 1996) imply that we are connected already through a variety of fields (e.g. electromagnetic, psychic, etc.). In such a reality, it is not necessary to become the other or move into their 'space'; instead, one interconnects through a kind of frequency attunement.

Husserl's ([1929]1967) intersubjectivity names a general field or ground of subjectivity that is also part of our individual subjectivity. He refers to the authentic meeting in that space as transcendental empathy. And as Rogers (1980) concludes, it is not so much a state as it is a process. Deep empathy is 'not a state of consciousness but an activity of awareness that can integrate states of consciousness' (Puhakka 2000). The duality of self and not-self shifts in such direct knowing into an intersubjective experience: what Thich Nhat Hanh (1995) calls 'interbeing', which refers to the fundamental connectedness of all things. Rogers (1980) describes this as follows: 'It seems that my inner spirit has reached out and touched the inner spirit of the other. Our relationship transcends itself and becomes part of something larger' (p. 129).

As attunement refines still further there is neither objective observation, nor seeing the world through the client's eyes, nor reacting to, nor fusing with, nor attuning to. Instead, the centre of perception seems to occupy multiple perspectives simultaneously. One seems to become the field itself while maintaining awareness, as there is less identification with the perspective from a single self or vantage point. Aurobindo writes: 'In order to see, you have to stop being in the middle of the picture' (cited in Nelson 1994: 311). This witnessing is often experienced with more emotional detachment. As an example, Myss (1996) describes her experiences as having the quality of 'impersonal daydreams' (p. 2). She suggests that 'their impersonality, the nonfeeling sensation of the impressions, is extremely significant' (p. 2), as an indicator of the epistemic process of receiving information.

Phenomenologically, information is often encountered as if it were coming from another source, perceived as outside or deep inside. This is similar to the phenomenon of inspiration (Hart 1998). Some describe this as tuning into the person's higher self that may be accomplished through asking oneself a simple question: 'How can I be of help to this person?' 'What should I be aware of?' Developmentally, this knowing may correspond to experiences of Rowan's (1993) Surrendered Self and probably to the late Psychic and early Subtle stages of Wilber's (1995) developmental model. As the therapist opens to this field of consciousness, other kinds of material become available (unexpected images, including possible archetypal themes, deep patterns, etc.) that may not be available to the client's immediate awareness. Empathic information may also arrive in literal or symbolic form. As an example, with one client a symbolic image emerged (before there was any content exchanged verbally) in which the paradox of the client's dilemma was represented as a leaf, frozen, which will shatter if it is touched but which remains lifeless if it is not. This aspect of the matter can be particularly helpful when working with clients from other cultures. Fukuyama and Sevig (1999) provide copious references to research on the transpersonal relationship in this area.

While one may hypothesize origins and infer patterns in more conventional empathy, in this level of refinement it becomes increasingly possible to recognize and appreciate multiple layers and patterns of experience intuitively and immediately. For example, the strong imagery and body sensations so rich and available at previous levels may be recognized as constructed phenomena or consequences that have roots in fundamental beliefs or patterns of thought. In this degree of empathic refinement, the therapist is less likely to be carried away emotionally as attention shifts from feelings and thoughts (although it can still include them) to more subtle and inclusive patterns that may underlie them.

Linking

One of us has suggested elsewhere (Rowan 1998b), following research by Budgell (1995), that we can subsume all these phenomena under the heading of 'linking'. Linking is that way of relating that refuses to take separation seriously, and assumes instead that the space between therapist and client can be fully occupied and used by both, to the advantage of the therapeutic work. This can only be done in a state of subtle consciousness where the fear of relating such a depth can be overcome or set aside or just not experienced.

Linking can be seen as a special kind of empathy, a special kind of countertransference or a special kind of identification. Various terms, some of which have already been referred to above, can be found to be examples of this phenomenon of linking, such as 'resonance', 'experiential listening', 'embodied countertransference', 'being aligned', 'working at relational depth', 'the four-dimensional state', 'the unifying I–Me relationship' and 'melding'. It is not a new therapy or a new technique, but simply recognition of a relatively unfamiliar human relationship, which has been formally researched and described in a number of sources.

Budgell describes 'linking' as:

> The experience is described as near fusion, a communion of souls or spirits and a blurring of personal boundaries. To achieve this, both parties have to give up something of themselves while remaining separate. It is not symbiosis but the other end of the spectrum, as described by Wilber (1980a). It is the transpersonal sense of relinquishing self. Symbiosis is about being cosy, but this is about working through pain and fear. It is a sacred experience and yet natural and there all the time. It comes from the spiritual or transpersonal realm, being a step beyond empathy and the natural plain.
>
> (Budgell 1995: 33)

Budgell found over and over again that therapists who had had these experiences did not want to reduce them to something which could be controlled. 'It was a sense of being joined or linked and of something good and healing emanating from another person' (Budgell 1995: 63). The essence of it was that it came unbidden.

Grof (1988) describes two closely related phenomena, 'dual unity' and 'identification with other persons', both of which involve the loosening or melting of the boundaries of the ego. Grof tells the story of his wife Christina 'moving inside' Gregory Bateson, who at the time lived nearby: she felt as if she were within him, and feeling everything he felt, even to the extent of knowing he was dying of cancer, which no one had said up to that point. Grof says: 'It seemed clear that experiences of this kind would be invaluable for diagnostic and therapeutic purposes, if they could be brought under full voluntary control' (Grof 1988: 49). This seems to be progressive rather than regressive and to represent something not dealt with in most texts.

Linking is a phenomenon which is to be found in Jungian, existentialist, humanistic and psychoanalytic writings. For example, Winnicott (1975) speaks many times of 'the third area', 'the intermediate area' and 'an area of freedom'. This is essentially between people, rather than inside either of them. In his thinking, it links closely with the concept of a transitional object, being the place where transitional objects are experienced. It appears, from our review of different descriptions of this type of experience, that linking is understood by some as arising spontaneously, while there is an element of being able to 'produce' it in the view of others. The idea, however described, needs a great deal more work.

Not knowing – an alternative view of the transpersonal?

We are aware that for some therapists the levels of work we describe here border on the mystical and perhaps even the bizarre. Certainly the experiences in therapy we describe are intellectually challenging, but no doubt emotionally challenging as well. Being with the client in this way involves the therapist in being ready to let go of concentration on the ego. He or she is able to move largely beyond what the transpersonal psychologist Wilber calls 'mental-ego consciousness' and also beyond what he calls 'Centaur consciousness'. This links up with two types of mystical experience, the parallels to which we referred to at the start of this chapter. While mysticism is generally associated with union with the divine or the transcendent, many of the references in this chapter have clearly described a type of union (albeit one which also recognizes separation) between therapist and client, one which appears to step beyond identification and similar terms examined in Chapter 3.

There is another expression of transcendent experience and of letting go of 'mental ego-consciousness' that is more commonly seen in Eastern mysticism, but with a representation in Western tradition, too. This often refers to transcendent experience through the language of negation. Put in Winnicott's terminology (although not expressed this way by Winnicott), this may suggest a *void* in the space between, rather than a space between therapist and client where there is linking. Bion refers to 'not knowing' (and one Western mystical tradition refers to unknowing): 'without memory or desire' (Bion 1970) may express this in relation to therapy itself. This more agnostic form certainly transcends (partially, or at least part of the time) all the ways of understanding the use of self in earlier chapters. There is recognition of an experience that cannot be expressed in words or images: we have referred above to Bion's use of the letter 'O' to encompass the experience, and Milner goes one stage further by using '0' (nought) when referring to Bion's 'O' (Milner 1987: 267–8). It is interesting to see how many psychoanalysts have touched on this idea, even if sometimes in a peripheral or glancing manner, as for example Winnicott, Eigen, Searles, Bollas, Grotstein, Stern, Kohut, Ferenczi and Balint.

Bion was very interested in the question of psychic reality. How does an analyst decide how and when to make an interpretation? Bion's answer is that it is through the process of intuition. This involves letting go of the senses. He likened it to the idea of Negative Capability as explained by John Keats. He writes: 'The capacity of the mind depends on the capacity of the unconscious – negative capability. Inability to tolerate empty space limits the amount of space available' (Bion 1992: 304). The term 'negative capability' describes the state of mind the analyst must strive for, like *reverie* (another of Bion's terms). This appears to be something more than Freud's injunction for the analyst to enter a state of 'free-floating attention', especially when the term is also used for the nursing mother's attention to her baby. Milner is similarly struck by Keats' phrase in looking at the significance of doubt and un-knowing in the psychoanalytic setting (Milner 1987: 260), while Britton (1998: 15) draws our attention to a footnote of Freud's in which Freud describes a state of mind as 'the blindness of the seeing eye [in which] one knows and does not know a thing at the same time' (Freud and Breuer 1895). Britton himself suggests 'that the *suspension of belief* is a non-psychotic form of disavowal in which one believes and does not believe a thing at the same time' (Britton 1998: 15, emphasis in original).

Here we have something that appears to be different from the transpersonal experience described above. In what we have described so far, there appears to be a state of mind that can be cultivated, even if the experience itself cannot be engineered, in which the therapist is more attuned to her or his responses (physical, emotional and intellectual) as they arise from the therapeutic relationship. Bion appears to be suggesting a type of *kenosis* (emptying) of the self, not a greater attunement of the self. Our defences protect us from 'the non-sensuous world of thought, because the pain . . . is felt to be intolerable' (Symington and Symington 1996: 182). Psychoanalysis, according to this view, is the investigation of such a relationship. It attempts to open both partners to this experience, which, like the working through pain and fear in Budgell's description above of transpersonal work, is an invitation to 'venture forth into the unknown and risk the terror' (Symington and Symington 1996: 184). Bion concentrates his focus on those elements that block the two individuals from that experience.

Bion is probably not a typical psychoanalyst, although he is looked upon with high esteem by many psychoanalysts and has to be taken seriously. It is also interesting to see him endorsing the concept of linking in the way he does, although his paper 'Attacks on linking' (Bion 1967) has a slightly different purpose: he describes the psychotic patient attacking the link between analyst and patient, trying to undermine the analyst's task of integrating the various elements in the patient's communications.

Winnicott, too, in philosophical mood, shows some uncertainty about whether we ever make direct contact with external reality – and, therefore, by implication, with another. This sounds strange coming from one who (see below) clearly made deep contact with many of those who were his patients. Nevertheless, he maintains that there is 'only an illusion of contact, a midway phenomenon that works very well for me when I am not tired' (Winnicott 1988: 114–15). He writes in the same context of 'the essential aloneness of the human being' (p. 144).

Some caveats

Winnicott's words may bring us up with a start. He appears in them to challenge the notion that the therapist makes deep contact with the client. Certainly, we have to acknowledge that there are other ways of looking at these experiences. What may be an illusion of moving deeper into the transpersonal might also be understood by some theorists as regression. Freud, with his devotion to the reality principle, understood such experiences generally as oceanic feelings and as a return to the mother–baby symbiosis. Wilber, as a transpersonal psychologist, has no doubt about transcendental experience, but cautions that sometimes it is more an indication of regression to the prepersonal (Wilber 1980b). Winnicott allowed some of his patients to regress to a boundaryless oneness with him so that the wounds of early trauma could be healed. One of those patients, Margaret Little (1990), also writes of regression, and says that the therapist at a certain point may have to allow the patient to enter the therapist's own inner world and become part of it. The therapist is possessed, for a longer or shorter time. It is essentially an adaptation to the needs of the patient at a particular time, but not a continuous activity in all therapeutic work. We have no doubt that this is something genuinely therapeutic, but might see this as prepersonal rather than transpersonal, in the sense that it reproduces something infantile or even foetal, or, as Little (1990) says, Winnicott's 'primary maternal pre-occupation' rather than Freud's 'free-floating attention' (p. 89). This is a very different type of linking, because it is regressive. Nevertheless, even if the distinction between pre- and transpersonal is a vital one, prepersonal experience is no more all bliss than transpersonal linking, and the therapist entering into this relationship with the patient may well have to experience what analysts call 'the paranoid-schizoid position'.

The other caveat is that we have to acknowledge that there are therapists who deny the whole idea of relationship; this, therefore, renders the idea of a relationship beyond the normal therapeutic one as more tenuous.

Conclusion

Perhaps the best way of summing up the third way of using the self in therapy is to say that it involves moving into an altered state of consciousness. That is the aspect of it which we may call Being. Having moved into that state of consciousness, which essentially partakes of what some would call the sacred, the numinous, the holy, we can then be more creative in our relationship with the client. We are as it were drawing on something bigger than both of us. Whatever techniques may emerge from this process will be uniquely suitable for the moment. This is the aspect of it which we may call Doing, and a good example of it is to be found in Maguire (2001). In carrying out this work, we may refer to any or all of the theorists mentioned above: this is the Knowing aspect. But another way of looking at Knowing is to say that the form of thought most useful at this level is intuition, considered here as something that comes from outside, and which in a way we do not own. We allow it rather than construct it. This raises the interesting question of how, if this level of use of self is accepted as valid, therapists can attain it. Can it be taught? Or does it have to be caught? This, and other questions about the instrumental self and the authentic self as related to training and supervision form the subject of the next chapter.

Training and supervision

There are obvious implications for training in the preceding chapters, although we realize that not everything we have discussed can be 'trained'. Some of the therapist's use of self, perhaps much of it, consists of qualities, not skills; and although qualities can be encouraged to grow, they can only be talked about or modelled by a trainer or a supervisor to a trainee. Similarly, the way therapists conduct themselves has its own impact upon clients: who the therapist is and the way the therapist relates may be as important as what the therapist says. It may be that in psychotherapy training and supervision, that we learn as much, for good or ill, from the milieu of a training course and from the manner of the supervision as we do from its content. Nevertheless, in this chapter we examine both the content of training and supervision, inasmuch as it applies to the therapist's use of self; as well as the implicit messages that are transmitted, which reinforce either conformity or originality in the way in which therapists regard themselves, in relation to their orientation and the qualifying body, as well as in turn to their clients.

In a paper of fascinating historical interest, Michael Balint (writing in 1948, about half-way through the period of the development of psychotherapy and counselling to date, between the singular work of Freud and the present multiplicity of approaches) observed that much of the discussion of training in psychoanalysis had up to that time been in secret, with very little committed to publication, unusual when the same influential figures discussing these matters were otherwise prolific in print! He regards the lack of public debate as indicative of inhibition, rather than lack of interest, and suggests that:

the whole atmosphere is strongly reminiscent of the primitive initiation ceremonies. On the part of the initiators – the training committee and the training analysts – we observe secretiveness about our esoteric knowledge, dogmatic announcements of our demands and the use of authoritative techniques. On the part of the candidates, i.e. those to be initiated, we observe the willing acceptance of the exoteric [*sic*] fables, submissiveness to dogmatic and authoritative treatment without much protest and too respectful behaviour. We know that the general aim of all initiation rites is to force the candidate to identify himself with his initiator, to introject the initiator and his ideals, and to build up from these identifications a strong super-ego which will influence him all his life.

(Balint 1948: 167)

We believe this is not just true of 1948, but also true of today (see below, particularly Kernberg's criticism of psychoanalytic training). We also believe it is not just true of psychoanalysis, but applies equally to other psychotherapeutic models. In this chapter, we wish both to examine models of training and question how best to develop the therapist's use of self. Balint indicates how any trainee, simply because he or she wishes to qualify in a profession (which today is even more regulated than then), may conform to what is laid down and expected, and so possibly diminish the development of their true self. Menzies (1960) has observed that, in a parallel profession, many nurses in training are obliged to collude with the primitive anxieties and defences of the institution in which they work, meaning restriction of their own personality. Indeed, Menzies found that the more mature students left the profession!

Training as a psychotherapist or counsellor usually involves three or four components: theoretical knowledge, the learning of technical skills, personal therapy and supervision. In some training (psychoanalysis, for example), the learning of technical skills is often assumed to come about through learning from one's own analyst and from supervision, and may not be a discrete area. In contrast to this, validation of courses by the British Association for Counselling and Psychotherapy has been insistent upon making the distinction between skills training and the teaching of theory, and requiring both.

Learning theory and therapeutic skills might be seen as equivalent to the first major theme of our own study: the self of the therapist as instrumental. Personal therapy may serve different purposes, according to one's view of the therapist's use of self. It may, for example, be undertaken to remove as much of the bias and extraneous influence of the trainee's own agenda from her or his practice to arrive at the maximum objectivity in relation to the client's material. Those who held (or hold) that countertransference was and is solely a negative influence upon practice clearly support personal training analyses as a means of modifying its significance. Those who believe in learning from one's own experience may see personal therapy as a means to model practice upon one's own therapist. At the very least, a therapist ought to experience what it is like to be a client. Those who hold that there is a vast commonality in the unconscious (i.e. that we are all, at least in the unconscious, made up of the same drives or share in the same characteristics in the internal world) may wish to extend personal therapy as being the most illuminating area of study. Others would claim that it is imperative that a therapist has gone as far as possible along the path of self-actualization.

Early views on training

One of the criticisms of Freud is that he never underwent a personal analysis. He relied on his self-analysis, supported by his correspondence with Fliess (Masson 1985), in which intense relationship Freud was able to find some relief from the isolation he experienced in delving into the unconscious – both his own and that of his patients. We need not doubt that this capacity to discuss his ideas continued in the many professional relationships and personal friendships that flowered as his ideas assumed greater significance, although it is difficult to know just how frank he was about his inner life. Critics have pointed to his refusal to discuss a particular dream with Jung, although Jones (1955) writes of Freud's correspondence with Jung as 'a most friendly and even intimate exchange of both personal thoughts as well as scientific reflections' (p. 35). This was the way things were in those early years. Jones' 'training analysis' with Ferenczi in 1913 was very brief, four months in all, and he was one of the first of the early analysts to be analysed. We know that they also discussed ideas alongside the personal analysis. Ferenczi's formal analysis with Freud consisted of just a few weeks in 1914 and in 1916 – and they were for many years very close friends as well. Ferenczi was later to criticize Freud for failing to analyse the negative transference (Dupont 1995: xiii), to which Freud's reply was that it did not at that time exist!

It was not until 1922 that the first clear rules for training emerge, when Eitingon in Berlin writes: 'We are all firmly convinced that henceforth no one who has not been analysed must aspire to the rank of practising analyst. It follows that the analysis of the student himself is an essential part of the curriculum and takes part at the Polyclinic in the second half of the training period, after a time of intensive theoretical preparation by lectures and courses of instruction'. (Today personal therapy is often seen as needing to start before 'courses of instruction'.) The average time of the whole training is given as one to one and a half years (Balint 1948: 165). By 1924 it was laid down in Berlin that the training analysis must last at least six months and the whole training is to last for about three years: the theoretical training needs a minimum of two terms and the control work a minimum of two years. Control work refers to the 'control analysis', the psychoanalytic terminology for 'supervised practice'.

There was a debate about whether the training analyst should also conduct the control analysis – that is, be the supervisor as well as the therapist – and there was recognition of the distinction between the countertransference in the student that formed part of the training analysis, and working with patients who may have very different problems from the student that was the basis for the control analysis. According to the Hungarian Institute, the analysis of the countertransference was best done if the training and the control analyses were carried out by the same person, at least with the first case; and in Hungary, too, there was a determined attack against the false conception of dividing the training into three independent parts. The debate continued without clear decisions, waiting for evidence on what was best, independent analyst and supervisor or the same person. Balint observes that, in 1947, London laid down the rule, 'The analyst undertaking the student's personal analysis does not undertake the supervision of his case', but that as far as he knew, this statement was not the result of carefully planned and controlled observations: 'it sounds to me like yet another dogmatic compulsory ruling' (Balint 1948: 166).

It is interesting that Aponte and Winter (2000: 132), writing from a humanistic perspective, say that it is uncommon to find a training model that consistently maintains a focus on both the conduct of therapy, with specific case interventions, and the practitioner's personal issues, and the interaction between the two. They urge that more attention to this matter is very important. They say: 'Assisting a therapist to incorporate his or her own personal qualities into technical interventions with clients is the core process in the use of self in therapy' (Aponte and Winter 2000: 132). It is possible to see some links here to ideas circulating in Hungarian psychoanalysis before the Second World War.

Balint makes it clear that, in the beginning, the form of training as an analyst was a matter of personal choice: how much personal analysis was left to analysand and analyst. And the choice of the training analyst was also personal, not laid down by a central authority. After the secessions of leading figures, it appears that more and more centralized control came into force – first from local training institutes and then laid down, at least in part, internationally. The third development, still happening when Balint wrote, was that the various factions within psychoanalysis sought to put their own stamp upon the training, part of which was done through supervision, or the control analysis. Balint comments, clearly not afraid of speaking his mind:

> There is ample opportunity during the training analysis to change an independent or indifferent candidate into a fervent proselyte. This danger increases with the control work. We know that the analyst is in fact introjected during analysis and used as a nucleus of a new super-ego; but what is introjected is an unrealistic image of the analyst, adapted by distortions to the patient's needs and subsequently subjected to a conscious correction during the period of working through. The balance of forces is quite different during the control situation.
>
> There the control analyst is a real person with strong convictions, theoretical likes and dislikes, preoccupations, and personal limitations. He is not bound by the analytical situation, he can – and often does – represent his views and convictions, with all his weight; moreover, the candidate has a much weaker stand in this situation, he has not the privilege of using his free associations – his strongest defence – any more, he is taught and controlled or 'supervised' not analysed. The balance of forces is somewhat different but by no means more favourable to the candidate in the lectures and seminars. Not only does the lecturer speak *ex cathedra*, but any contradiction immediately singles out the candidate, who from then on has to face a conformist group as a non-conformist individual, a strain to which only a few can and dare stand up.
>
> (Balint 1948: 170–1)

Balint (1948: 171) notes that 'the two great masters of analytic technique, Freud and Ferenczi, did not take a prominent part in this kind of training. Somehow they seemed to be satisfied with analysis only'.

Personal therapy

Freud (1937) acknowledged 'that analysts do not in their own personalities wholly come up to the standards of psychic normality which they set for their patients', and suggested that to try and remedy this analysts should be re-analysed every five years, a suggestion that was never taken up. Ferenczi and Rank (1925) urged that the training analysis should be deeper and more thorough than the therapeutic analysis usually is. It appears from the literature that to begin with there was little clarity about the function of the training analysis. Mainly it was to remove 'blind spots'. But as training analysts themselves developed their understanding of their function, the purpose broadened. Benedek, herself one of the pioneers who had only a cursory training analysis, describes how as a supervisor she learned more of what was required in a training analysis. She had not only a therapeutic aim, but was also preparing the candidate to be an analyst. In the early years, this was done through the didactic element of the training analysis, 'instructional analysis' as it was sometimes called. But Benedek writes in 1969, some fifty years after her own training:

> The training analyst is entrusted with developing the student's capabilities to function as an instrument of the analytic process . . . He assesses not only the developmental conflicts and the personality of the student, but also his perceptiveness, his communication with his unconscious, his empathy and his 'humanity', as well as his endurance for the empathic understanding of that humanness which continually requires his productive, helpful response.
>
> (Benedek 1969: 442)

In contrast to the paucity of open communication about training in the first thirty years of psychoanalysis, there is a fair spread of articles on training appearing in the psychoanalytic journals, despite the complaint in some of them that little is publicly written still on these questions. Differences between continents and major training institutes are apparent, especially in the various reports of the major psychoanalytic conferences, to which we shall return below for comments on the critique of training (Wallerstein 1978, 1988,

1993). Training is actively debated and even reviewed by students in training (e.g. Bruzzone *et al.* 1985). One of the central topics is the reporting or non-reporting of the personal analysis by the training analyst: practice differs in various countries on this. For example, writing in 1982, Sandler describes the training analyst in the UK as being required to report every six months, until the student takes her or his first case. The training analyst has to agree to the student starting theory seminars and taking their first clinical cases. But reports are generally brief, without having to go into detail. In Denmark, the responsibility for reporting shifts, after the student has started theoretical seminars, from training analyst to supervisor.

Obviously these requirements change from time to time. There is general agreement in the literature that the dual function of the training analyst, being simultaneously a therapist and a teacher and an assessor of progress, may seriously hamper the training analysis, including the degree of confidences that the student can share with the analyst. Unless there can be a totally non-judgemental relationship it is impossible, it is argued, for the student to make full use of the requirement of analysis for free association. There are clearly some institutes where it is accepted that the training analyst does not have to report, and where the only real concern is how to deal with a situation when a candidate clearly has the type of problems that cast doubt on the ability to practise.

There is debate, too, about what a training analysis should achieve: what makes it 'good enough'? Fleming and Weiss (1978) list the following criteria, where the order of the items is worth noting, as well as their emphasis on personal qualities and personal knowledge, rather than upon academic knowledge and its application to practise:

1 It will have developed the candidate's potential for empathic understanding and communication with self and others.
2 It will have provided a first-hand, very personal experience in learning about unconscious conflict, anxiety, resistance, defence, symptomatic behaviour (such as learning blocks), genetic determinants, dreams, regression and transference.
3 It will have developed skill in introspecting, associating and interpreting latent meanings, all relevant for continuing self-analysis.
4 It will have developed some insight into the conflicts that have played a major role in determining the candidate's character structure and neurotic symptoms.

5 It will have developed some insight into the Oedipus conflict in particular and how the candidate has resolved.

(Fleming and Weiss 1978: 36)

Sedgwick (1993: 120–1), comparing Jung and Searles, states that both men look to a training analysis for a refinement of the therapist's personality, so as to be able to use it in therapy. Just to react to patients is too cavalier. Searles and Jung both stress the person rather than the method and both stress the need for personal analysis. Neither believes that the unconscious will be fathomed, but that therapists will be less tainted by their own projections and will have a more accurate perception of unconscious feeling processes. 'What he is really developing is a subjectivity he can trust' (Sedgwick 1993: 121). Indeed:

> the primary value of a training analysis, in its aspect of equipping the analytic candidate to function effectively as an analyst, consists in helping him to become sufficiently in touch with his own emotional life so that when one or another area of this is evoked in his work with a patient he can feel sufficiently at ease with it to remain interested in discerning what subtle but real processes at work in the patient, heretofore unanalyzed, have provided the stimulus for this evocation.
>
> (Searles *et al.* 1973: 358)

Searles (1955) acknowledges, and indeed is not over-concerned, that self-awareness can never be so complete as to free a therapist from emotional involvement, particularly when there is a high degree of anxiety in the client. Similarly, from the Jungian tradition, the purpose of training analysis is not merely to heal the personality of the analyst, but to open his wounds from which his compassion will flow – here the concept of the wounded healer (see p. 59) is relevant (Hillman 1973/1990: 132).

In humanistic approaches, personal therapy is equally essential. 'Training for becoming more fully human' is one of the phrases used by Satir, according to Lander and Nahon (2000: 10): 'Being this kind of self-actualized person is a necessary prerequisite that enables one human being to reach out in healthy ways to another with the kind of fidelity and consistency on which trust is built in the healing context'. There is some evidence for the circular idea that acceptance of others is based on acceptance of one's self, and that self-acceptance is based largely on being accepted by others. Several early studies (Sherman 1945; Phillips 1951; Zelen 1954) point to the significance of self-acceptance and other positive self-regarding attitudes as basic for acceptance of others. The significance of these findings for personal therapy is obvious. There is also recognition of the needs of the therapist and that these should not be met solely through being a therapist.

It appears that most orientations, therefore, make it a condition of training that there should be an element of personal therapy or, as it is called in some humanistic traditions, personal growth and development. Cognitive-behavioural psychotherapy is different, and the UK Council for Psychotherapy arrived at a tactful form of words for them, which specified that all members had to arrive at arrangements to ensure that the trainees can identify and manage appropriately their personal involvement in and contributions to the processes of the psychotherapies that they practise. What this amounts to in practice is the use of supervision, which is compulsory for all members of the Behavioural and Cognitive Psychotherapy Section of the UK Council for Psychotherapy. It appears that supervision is not just used for technical corrections, but also for the further development of the person of the therapist. The advantage in practising techniques first-hand has been suggested by Padesky (1996) and 'in the case of behaviour therapy it would clearly be an advantage to overcome a personal phobia before treating a client with a similar difficulty' (Ricketts and Donohoe 2000: 131). However, it is obviously better to employ supervision widely and deeply rather than expect these kinds of coincidences. Clinical psychologists have also had no requirement for personal therapy, but it is necessary for chartered counselling psychology status through the British Psychological Society. This may make for an interesting dialogue if and when membership of the two sections becomes interchangeable.

The main difference between the orientations has to do with frequency and length of personal therapy, in line with the assumptions made about the necessary requirements for therapy itself. In the psychoanalytic schools, anything less than twice weekly personal therapy, before and throughout training, is frowned upon, and is one of the main differences in Britain between the British Confederation of Psychotherapists representing the stricter requirements and the UK Council for Psychotherapy.

Most courses, therefore, require students to be in therapy, even if they differ on how many hours are required. Nevertheless, there are questions about this which some of the humanistic schools (particularly the person-centred) raise more obviously, on the grounds that personal therapy needs to be congruent with where a person is in their self-development. One argument, therefore, is that the student should seek therapy when he or she feels the need for it, otherwise entering therapy is artificial. There is also a challenge from research that shows that therapists who have received personal counselling are no more effective (Feltham and Dryden 1993: 134; Russell 1993); and even research cited from various sources that has 'established' that much counselling and psychotherapy training has a detrimental effect, both on the trainees and the distressed members of the public they would like to help (Dineen 1996). Although we would not take this view ourselves and would want to challenge this research, we nevertheless recognize the value of this type of argument, and can see how it might also be argued, from a less extreme position, that the length, frequency and choice of personal therapy for students and practitioners should ideally be dictated by the individual in dialogue with their therapist, and that this part of the training should be kept distinct from other aspects of assessment.

The dynamics of supervision

We have already alluded to the question in the preliminary schemes for training in analysis as to whether the student's therapist and supervisor should be the same person. In arguing for this, Kovacs (1936) makes it clear that in those days (at least in Hungary) the trainee did not begin the control analysis (supervised practice) until his or her personal analysis was over. Kovacs argues for the same analyst and supervisor on the grounds that when the trainee begins to see patients, a whole new set of personal issues arise:

> If the candidate continues his own analysis when he begins to analyse patients, the two parallel pieces of work bring to light those sides of his personality which have hitherto received too little attention or none at all, or at least could not manifest them-selves in so expressive a fashion. All his good and bad qualities, and also his weaknesses, are revealed; for example, his incapa-city for objectivity; his impatience; his vanity; his inability to bear criticism; the tendency to observe only what is in his favour and the failure to note the serious accusations which the patient is bringing against him but dares not express except in a disguised form; the tactlessness which ministers to those sadistic or masochistic instincts in himself which he has failed

to master; his callousness or, on the other hand, his exaggerated
fellow-feeling and excessive tolerance.

(Kovacs 1936: 351–2)

This is a rather fine definition of the purpose of supervision, although by 1955 Searles describes supervision in analytic training
as limited 'mainly to . . . carefully listening to the therapist's verbal
report and making suggestions regarding improved handling of the
material which the patient has been producing' (Searles 1955: 157).
Supervision was purely an intellectual discussion, into which the
use of the self – whether the feelings of the supervisee or those of
the supervisor – were essentially an intrusion. At that time, there
was recognition that feelings such as rivalry could interfere with the
supervisory process, but such feelings were seen only in terms of
transference in the supervisee or countertransference within the
supervisor. This is analogous to the first level of the therapist's use
of self: that the function of supervision is promoting the skills and
knowledge of the therapist in relation to the patient's material, re-
fining the therapist in her or his instrumental use of the self. This
function is reflected in the process, which is largely didactic, even
though some supervisors encourage the self-supervision of the therapist in similarly reflecting upon the material.

We might argue that there are different levels of supervision as
there are different notions of the use of the self in therapy. Supervision might be seen as about correction, spontaneity or meditation.
The supervisee at the first level, similar to our description of the use
of self in Chapter 2, is seen as a learner technician, who has to be
helped to improve in technique and, in some schools, in rooting
theory in practice. The supervisor is seen as an educator more than
as a counsellor or facilitator (Carroll 1996: 27), sometimes teaching
skills in a well-defined way, quite concretely (Forsyth and Ivey 1980:
246). Model application and even model building will be a focus.
Lidmila (1997) suggests that the supervisor at this level may behave
like a detective, an inquisitor or a librarian.

The supervisor evaluates the supervisee and corrects any tendencies to deviate from good practice (Holloway 1995: 3). Similarly, the
supervisee is regarded as someone who has to be carefully watched
and kept in line. Monitoring is felt to be a major concern. A single
model of the therapeutic process is generally favoured.

In psychodynamic supervision at this level, according to the
classic work of Ekstein and Wallerstein (1972), it is understood that
the supervisory experience is often inhibited by intrapsychic conflicts

and resistances in the student and occasionally in the supervisor. It is believed that the primary commitment of the supervisor should be directed towards the patient, in keeping with the principle espoused by Langs (1980), that once a physicianly responsibility is established on any level, it takes precedence over all else. Within this level, a great deal of importance is given to the unconscious, but the depth to which the unconscious is plumbed makes no difference to the level on which the work is practised, since it is the unconscious of the patient more than the unconscious of the therapist that is under consideration. Indeed, some psychoanalytic supervisors would insist that any material coming from the therapist should be taken back into the therapist's personal therapy. The main focus is often on the client and on the supervisee's relationship with the client.

In cognitive-behavioural work at this level, as Wessler and Ellis (1980) have argued, supervisors try to remain especially alert to times when supervisees agree with their clients' irrational beliefs, thereby becoming co-sufferers; and when they help their clients avoid rather than work on their disturbances. Clarity about aims is a major value. There is a great emphasis upon skills. The early training initiatives sought 'theoretical congruence of treatment models and supervisory approaches, with the directive, educational aspects of therapy providing a model for supervisory interventions' (Ricketts and Donohoe 2000: 129). According to Fruzzetti *et al.* (1997), in dialectical behaviour therapy supervision moves from 'a therapy skills acquisition phase' to 'skill application with individual clients' (p. 86). Some trainers in this area seem only to see the whole question as a matter of skills, distinguishing for example between the mere identification of skills, through basic mastery of skills, to active mastery of skills, all the way up to teaching skills to others (Daniels *et al.* 1997). Others merely seem to assume that skills are primary because they can be measured and tested (Kratochwill *et al.* 1997).

The basic goals of therapy supervision at this first level, regardless of therapeutic orientation, are to assist the therapist both to do effective therapy in the present and to achieve the capability to carry out effective therapy independent of the supervisor (Linehan 1980: 149). There may be a good deal of challenging of the supervisee. There is thus an emphasis on competence and doing what is correct, and making sure that both supervisor and supervisee do not stray too far from good practice. When the supervisee gets it right, there may be praise and confirmation. There is a good deal of attention to being helpful and getting good results. There is little interest in the social or political aspects of the work, and what there is tends to be restricted to established political parties or single-issue campaigns. It is perhaps not surprising that this type of supervision is seen essentially as training, and as an activity that may be dropped as soon as the trainee qualifies, except for occasional consultation over difficult cases. It is interesting that despite the strictness over most aspects of the work, psychoanalytic trainings on the whole espouse a less rigorous model of supervision than humanistic or cognitive-behavioural trainings, regarding supervision as largely confined to the training period, with no requirement for ongoing regular supervision unless the therapist particularly chooses to want it.

The use of self in supervision

We may be unfair to identify the instrumental emphasis of supervision with the psychoanalytic and the cognitive-behavioural orientations. Certainly there has been a major shift in the perception of the supervisory process in psychoanalytic thinking, which is analogous to the shift in the perception of countertransference (Heimann 1950; see pp. 30–1). It occurred about the same time, in the 1950s, signalled by the classic paper by Searles on the emotional experiences of the supervisor in supervision. Having reviewed the tendency for supervision to be seen as an intellectual exercise, and for feelings in the therapist or supervisor to be viewed as transference or countertransference, Searles suggests an additional element which may be present: 'When a supervisor notices any certain feeling in himself, this, taken by itself, might be an indication of something primarily in *himself*, . . . or of something primarily so in the *therapist*, or of some area of difficulty primarily in the *patient*' (Searles 1955: 159, emphasis in original). This idea was later taken up and amplified in the 'seven-eyed supervision' model of Hawkins and Shohet (2000). It is a tentative paper, despite convincing examples, where Searles considers the different possibilities for understanding 'disturbances' in supervision. But his idea has caught on so greatly that the phrase 'parallel process' in relation to supervision is to be found not only in much psychodynamic literature, but also further afield in humanistic writing too. Indeed, parallel process has become so popular in the jargon that it is tempting to see it everywhere, although in fact such a widespread appeal to parallel process both weakens the concept and also masks therapist and supervisor ineptitude (see Jacobs 1996).

Searles, whom we have already cited as writing that therapists can and indeed perhaps should never be free from emotional reactions, argues for the capacity of the supervisor to be in touch with her or his own countertransference. Unresolved problem areas in the supervisor's life at least to some extent probably underlie the supervisor's emotional reactions, otherwise the reactions would not occur in so noticeable a fashion. In other words, it is our own neurosis that helps us understand the client better – once again we might refer to the Jungian idea of the wounded healer.

If we now move on to the second level of supervision, which parallels Chapter 3 in relation to the therapist's use of self, supervision can operate over and above the instrumental. In the humanistic schools, we find that creativity, or the ability to make effective personal changes, is regarded as very important and can be seen as starting with the freedom to use supervision to explore. Spontaneity is regarded as important in the supervision as it is in the therapeutic work itself. The vision of the supervisee is regarded as very important. There is a continual questioning of narrowness. The body is included; the social system is included; the family of origin is included; traumatic experience is included; different kinds of relationship are included. There is an experiential and holistic approach. The goal is seen, certainly by Beier and Young (1980), as helping the supervisee in the work of encouraging the client to question and vary his or her routines and accept the uncertainty which is a by-product of interpersonal exploration. Questioning rather than acceptance is what is asked of the supervisee. Confrontation may become very important if the supervisee becomes too passive or uncreative.

At this level, particularly within the humanistic tradition, supervision is often seen as a containing and enabling process, rather than an educational or therapeutic process. To be effective, it must be exploratory (Page and Wosket 1994: 39). This is because it is believed that for both supervisor and supervisee there is the basic growth motivation, a push towards differentiation, authenticity and new experience (Rice 1980: 138). The growth and development of the supervisee is most important. Above all, as the classic integrative text by Hawkins and Shohet (2000) makes clear, supervision is a place where both parties are constantly learning; and to stay a good supervisor is to continually return to question, not only the work of the supervisee, but also what the supervisor is doing and how he or she does it. Houston (1995: 95), from the gestalt perspective, asks the question: Is the supervisor taking the supervisee forward at the right pace towards self-confidence based on reality, and towards abundance motivation?

What is regarded as central is not education or correction or monitoring, but as Rioch and her colleagues insist, increased self-awareness both for supervisor and supervisee (Rioch *et al.* 1976: 3). There is little emphasis on correct technique, or the precision of one theory. It is more important for supervisor and supervisee both to be fully present in the supervision session, because this will help to enable the therapist to be fully present with the client in the therapy session. There is frequently an emphasis on integration and/or eclecticism. Often the question of aims is deliberately disregarded or de-emphasized; aims tend to be long-term rather than short-term. Simplicity is encouraged. The main focus is on the supervisee rather than on the client. A peer relationship is aimed at as the ultimate goal. The responsibility and authority for the consultation work of supervision are shared by supervisor and supervisee (Yontef 1997: 155).

Given this dimension to supervision, it is understandable that humanistic schools insist on regular ongoing supervision or consultancy. The term 'supervision' itself is sometimes objected to as indicative of the superiority of the supervisor: it is interesting that Searles (1962) also, from a psychoanalytic perspective, comments that the 'potential usefulness' of the supervisor comes not from being more intelligent or more effective as a practitioner than the supervisee, but from being 'at a greater psychological distance . . . from the patient's psychopathology . . . This greater distance leaves me relatively free from anxiety and able, therefore to think relatively clearly and unconstrictedly' (p. 587).

An equally favoured method among humanistic practitioners is the peer review group, who meet together at regular intervals to discuss cases and work on their reactions to clients of various kinds. Due to the wealth of experience available, a great deal of learning can take place. The 'peer group supervision' model is described by Fizdale (1958) and Watson (1973). The group members need to be mature and at the same general level of competence. In addition, they have to respect each other professionally and be interested in improving their own skills. A good discussion of this whole area is to be found in Aponte and Lyons (1980) and in Houston (1995). The work can be done at various levels, from the most didactic to the most feeling-oriented. On the whole, it is found that more trust builds up in the group if it is allowed to be more feeling-oriented when appropriate. But it is important for each member to insist on getting the form of feedback that is most useful for him or her personally. This is the approach of the Independent Practitioners Network, as described by House and Totton (1997) – these therapists refuse to join the UK Council for Psychotherapy, for reasons which are explained by Mowbray (1995). Another method, mutual supervision in a pair, is sometimes called the collegial-peer approach and is well described by Hess (1980).

The transpersonal in supervision

Moving on now to the third level, which was the subject of Chapter 4, there can be in supervision a focus not only on transpersonal material, but also on a transpersonal process. There is considerable emphasis on the further development and 'enlargement' of the supervisee. This includes encouraging her or his subtle perception and intuition. J.L. Henderson (1995: 156) proposes that the supervisee may need further education in the whole field of mythology and of archetypes, as part of the work of developing the ability to use the superconscious in therapy. It could also be said at this level, as James (1996) suggests, that the supervisory situation is a *temenos*, a sacred space within which transformation may take place. It might be said that when a therapist comes for supervision, he or she is going on retreat. Therapists come to stop and listen, to open their awareness: the supervisor is providing the space for retreat, the holding for retreat and the transpersonal context for retreat (Whitmore 1999: 3). The supervisor is responsible for the integrity of the container within which the therapist may be transformed; and the supervisor, like the therapist, is a wounded healer.

The whole interaction may be seen in archetypal terms. At any one moment in time, as Clarkson (1998: 143) writes, any supervisor may need to be a Cerberus guarding the territories and boundaries, or a Psyche-sorter of the wheat and barley of primary and secondary realities, or a Zeus-like referee between warring internal or external factions, or a Chironic mentor teaching and modelling the skills of healing, or even a Hestian flame of spiritual direction. Beebe (1995: 103) feels that the trickster archetype may certainly become involved in the double existence of the therapist being healer and healed at the same time. Brookes (1995: 122) has pointed out that the supervisor may need to encourage the therapist to educate the client in confronting the numinous and archetypal layers of their own experience. Corbett (1995: 75) observes that numinosity, like transference, may not be noticed until it is drawn to the therapist's attention. It should also be noted, as Cobb (1997: 275) has critically suggested, that many schools of therapy teach therapists how to run sessions with clients in such a way that they actually prevent any incursion of the sublime.

From these observations, we can see that instead of a focus exclusively on the personal aspects of the transference, the supervisor will also be interested in its archetypal aspects. There is a deep interest in how the Self manifests itself in the therapeutic field (Corbett 1995: 70), or how it may be seen in shamanic terms. Some supervisors believe that the shaman is the original expression of the archetypal intent in human society, but that over time some aspects of the shaman's identity have split off and developed a character and autonomy of their own (e.g. Henderson 1998: 65). From this kind of imaginal perspective, the significance of fantasy is discovered not so much through analysing or unmasking it, as through elaboration and following its lead. In other words, fantasy is treated less as an object of suspicion and more as a resource to be tapped, and this is true whether we are talking about individual or group therapy (Maclagan 1997: 63).

Analysis may be regarded as a mysticism of persons – and hence polyvalent, pluralistic, many-headed, many-bodied. Sometimes it is found that it is helpful for both supervisor and supervisee to have a personal mindfulness-awareness meditation practice, as has also been suggested before a therapy session, although this is not absolutely necessary (Rabin and Walker, undated). In the light of some of the cross-cultural material, prayer before the session may be indicated for some people – again both client and therapist. The supervisor might on occasion want to suggest this. It has been pointed out that there is a particular role for the transpersonal therapist in the field of cross-cultural work, because of the increased respect for all religious experiences that comes with transpersonal development. The research paper by Cinnirella and Loewenthal (1999), for example, shows that members of communities such as white Christian, Pakistani Muslim, Indian Hindu, orthodox Jewish and African Caribbean Christian have many different attitudes to counselling and psychotherapy, which makes some of them particularly suspicious of western types of therapy. The supervisor's role in this can be to encourage the transpersonal therapist to look for such experience and to make his or her presence known to the relevant people.

What we see here, therefore, is an awareness of the spiritual context within which in transpersonal practice all supervision takes place. The notion of the greater Self as opposed to the individual self is often stressed.

As the Jungian writer Samuels has insisted, the 'Mundus Imaginalis' should be given due weight in the thinking of both supervisor and supervisee. This is the imaginal world so well described by the Sufi scholar Henry Corbin (Samuels 1997: 158–64). Supervision can partake of this character, involving the 'superconscious'. At this level, intuition ceases to be a matter of chance, but instead becomes the primary way in which one thinks. It implies a regular opening up to contact with the divine, the sacred, which may then be experienced as an initiation (Henderson 1995: 157–8). Paradoxically, this involvement with the transcendent can also lead to interest in the social and political context, as Samuels (1993) has also suggested, where concern tends to be towards the long-term good, rather than towards briefer campaigns.

It is sometimes felt, certainly by Whitmore, that supervision from a transpersonal context requires an act of will on the part of the supervisor, to affirm that all supervision begins with the supervisor's internal state of consciousness and a commitment to work from the 'inside out', before even meeting the supervisee. This is a contrary attitude to 'outside in', where the supervisor is regarded as the expert and as doing something to the supervisee (Whitmore 1999: 1).

The process is therefore crucial, but there are areas that transpersonal supervision may from time to time hold expertise, which is either lacking, or alternatively explained, in other theoretical models. This can be described as the area of 'spiritual emergency' (Bragdon 1988; Grof and Grof 1990). Certain difficulties can arise when people move into the transpersonal area and are exposed to spiritual experiences for which they are not ready. It is important at these points not to see the solution in terms of psychiatry or the mental hospital. Christina and Stanislav Grof (1990) outline ten specific problems that can come out of such events:

1 Peak experiences.
2 Kundalini energy awakening: the energy of the charkas.
3 Near-death experiences.
4 Past-life memories.
5 Opening to life myth: a journey to the centre, to the central meaning of life.
6 Shamanic crisis, often involving a visit to the underworld, annihilation and rebirth.
7 Psychic opening: paranormal phenomena; out-of-body experiences.

8 Channelling: spirit guides, with the danger of ego inflation.
9 UFO encounters.
10 Possession, by an entity which may be good or evil.

The Grofs firmly believe that 'when the person is given an opportunity to confront and express the disturbing energy in a supportive and understanding setting, a profound spiritual experience often results, one that has an extraordinary healing and transformative potential' (Grof and Grof 1990: 99). Not quite in the same category, but offering the same kind of disconcerting experience, is cross-cultural work, which may involve discarnate entities of one kind and another, ranging from gods and goddesses to demons and devils, ghosts and witches. A great deal of fear may be aroused by such material for the client, and may be experienced similarly by a therapist who is not well versed in this area. The text by Fukuyama and Sevig (1999) can help with such issues. Transpersonal therapists are better able to handle this material than most other therapists, because of their experience of this third level of working, and the transformations of consciousness stand them in good stead (Wilber *et al.* 1986).

The three different levels of supervision that we have distinguished can be set out, as they are in Table 5.1, to highlight the differences between them. They can, however, be understood as co-existing, in the manner of Russian dolls, rather than as completely superseding one another. In other words, every transpersonal supervisor has also available to them the earlier formations and abilities. Every authentic supervisor has also available to them the techniques of the instrumental level. Each level has an important part to play in supervision. If a trainee simply does not know a certain technique, and the supervisor considers that it would fit very well with a certain problem, there is no reason why a supervisor at any level should not mention it. If the trainee has made an obvious mistake and is blind to that, a supervisor at any level has to make a decision as to what to do about it. The manner might be different; the language might be different; but the problem still needs to be tackled. There is, however, a caveat. Neither a therapist nor a supervisor can jump levels at will. It is impossible to work at the authentic level unless this has been discovered, either through personal therapy or through personal experience, or a combination of the two. Neither is it possible to become a transpersonal supervisor without engaging with the transpersonal for oneself. For many therapists and supervisors, there are some huge challenges in what we describe, as well as vast opportunities.

Table 5.1 The three levels of supervision

Level	Instrumental	Authentic	Transpersonal
Self	I am defined by others	I define who I am	I am defined by the Other(s)
Motivation	Need	Choice	Allowing
Personal goal	Adjustment	Self-actualization	Contacting
Social goal	Socialization	Liberation	Extending
Process	Healing – ego-building	Development – ego-extending	Opening – ego-reduction
Type of helper	Physician Analyst	Growth facilitator Wounded healer	Advanced guide Aware of self
Representative approaches	Hospital treatment Chemotherapy Some Ps-Anal. Directive Behaviour modification Cognitive-behavioural Some TA Crisis work REBT Brief therapy	Primal integration Some Ps-Anal. Open encounter Psychodrama Gestalt therapy Bodywork therapies Some transpersonal approach Person-centred Co-counselling Regression Experiential therapy Focusing	Psychosynthesis Some Jungians Some pagans Transpersonal Voice dialogue Some wicca or magic Psychospiritual Some astrology Some tantra Shamanism Zen therapy Four-dimensional
Focus	Individual and group	Group and individual	Supportive Community
Research methods	Qualitative and quantitative	Action research Collaborative	Transformative Mindful
Questions	Dare you face the challenge of the unconscious?	Dare you face the challenge of freedom?	Dare you face the loss of your boundaries?
Key issues	Acceptability Respect	Autonomy Authenticity	The numinous Imaginal vision

Learning theoretical perspectives

While we have concentrated upon personal therapy and supervision, we do not neglect the importance that a theoretical perspective has on the way in which the therapist works: it is after all a theory, a set of meanings attached to human behaviours, relationships and emotions that informs the perception of the therapist, and the way the therapist interprets her or his own experience with the client. We have already demonstrated how most schools insist that it is hard for a therapist to deal with something in the client that the therapist has not yet dealt with in his or her own therapy. The personal therapy element of training is limited by the theoretical perspective of the orientation in which the candidate is training, which may include – depending to a large extent upon the openness of the teacher to other theories – the ability or inability to appreciate perspectives which other orientations regard as vital.

As an example, the psychoanalytically trained Malan (1979: 164–70) deals with a case history where there are (to the humanistic therapist) clear signs of umbilical affect. The material is about tubes and starvation and all the rest of the phenomena, which Lake (1980) has described so well. In the view of the primal therapist, the patient is remembering life in the womb and a traumatic experience that happened there. Malan says that the experiences link firmly with *feeding at the breast* (his italics), and that 'any reference to an umbilical cord cannot be anything other than psychological anachronism'. Because Malan has, presumably, never been into this area in his own therapy, and because there appears to be no place for this in his own theory, he is compelled to understand the reference from his own perspective and, therefore (from a different perspective), he falsifies it.

Such examples can be found in other orientations as well, as the reader will know from reading outside their usual theoretical stance. Some therapists are psychologically open to other models and are particularly open to learn from their clients. Some are not. This has mainly been true about the experience of birth and the traumas resulting from it that affect clients' lives in many ways; but most therapists of all persuasions have never experienced this in their own work on themselves, and so when the client brings it up, from the perspective of therapies that recognize the significance of prenatal experience, he or she is not understood.

The same is true of transpersonal therapies that point to the fact that not only have most therapists not been through their own (probably psychotic) material in the womb and the birth process, but also they have not been through their own (probably mystical) material in the transpersonal level of development. And so they are, in the opinion of transpersonal therapists, going to falsify this material, too. If a client brings up such material he or she is going to be diverted into a channel with which the therapist is more familiar. All therapists understand the value of referral to a specialist on occasion, and we are pointing here to areas in which this might be considered useful to the client.

A further factor, which touches on epistemology and is not within the brief of this book, is different levels of knowledge. For example, much training involves the imparting of information that can too easily be absorbed undigested and treated as authoritative, without always being supported by personal experience or insight. We consider some of the dangers implicit in training below. The development of therapists moving in the direction of personal knowledge, rather than reliance on 'sacred' texts, thus becomes more authentic. Knowledge becomes more like Bion's symbol 'K' – 'getting to know' – rather than 'knowing'. At what might be thought in some schools to be the transpersonal level, but in others even beyond any orientation, there is 'unknowing', or Bion's symbol 'O' where, as Bion writes, psychoanalysis is 'a stripe on a tiger', part of larger reality (Eigen 1998: 17; for a more extensive treatment of levels of knowledge from a psychodynamic perspective, see Jacobs 2000a).

There are obvious implications here for training. Although we recognize that trainings cannot cover every facet in every orientation, those that are limited solely to their own theoretical stance, if they dismiss other schools as 'wrong', do a disservice to their trainees and to their patients, as well as to a truly academic approach to theory. There are weaknesses in any single approach: psychoanalysis is bound to a particular technique; humanistic theory is not good on countertransference, particularly negative countertransference; the cognitive-behavioural approach has had a strong bias against the unconscious. All three are weak on the transpersonal, and the transpersonal in turn can be weak on grounding, becoming too fascinated with the archetypal and the imaginative. There is much to be said for a more integrative training. Training historically has been very narrow.

There are also implications for supervision. Supervision, too, can have a greater set of interpretations to draw upon, making a huge difference to the form and content of the supervision. Similarly, continuing professional development can take on different perspectives, providing the opportunity not only for more depth but also more breadth after formal training has ceased. It is, of course, not too hard to refer to other facets at an intellectual level, but the rest of the person needs to be involved, too; and it may well be that full appreciation of the theoretical differences in other orientations cannot be reached without some personal experience of their therapy as well. It is easier to get a taste of cognitive-behavioural therapy, or the humanistic therapies, than it is of full-blown psychoanalysis. But at least if a therapist's primary training has been open, and their personal therapy has enabled continuing working upon the self, then the chances of absorbing other knowledge and viewing personal experience from another perspective is possible.

Training and supervision: conformity or self-actualization?

Training has not been much of an issue until recently. Training institutes just went on doing what they have been doing since their inception. Traditions formed rapidly and seamlessly – and exclusively. Each one tended to think theirs was the best, or even the only way of going on. There was a kind of sleepy sense of normality, or worse – the danger of only accepting those who conformed.

This has been most expressively stated in the one orientation that the outsider imagines might be the most rigorous and the least open to internal criticism, psychoanalysis. In Britain, the outspoken R.D. Laing (Mullan 1995: 143–71) and David Cooper (1967), and the more reserved Rycroft (1968, 1985) and Lomas (1973; King 1999), are all examples of critics of psychoanalytical training and of the pressure to conform to one set of techniques. The American and the international psychoanalytic journals are more extensively searching. We have referred above to differences in detail of requirements for training in various national institutes. In a presidential address to the International Psychoanalytic Association, Wallerstein (1988) commented on the 'increasing psychoanalytic diversity, or pluralism as we have come to call it, a pluralism of theoretical perspectives, of linguistic and thought conventions, of distinctive regional, cultural, and language emphases', and in a number of his many papers he draws together some of these differences. His 1993 paper summarizing the Fifth Conference of Training Analysts is a fascinating overview of this pluralistic position, as in his citing of one contributor who used the image of the 'inevitably Procrustean nature of orthodoxy in teaching and training with all the tendencies to rigidity and ideological indoctrination, to stretching or shortening our candidates to fit our mould, as against the Promethean analytical "youthful ardour" with perhaps its unconquerable creativity but also its inevitable mistakes and risks' (Wallerstein 1993: 165). Speakers ranged from the most conservative (a Swiss analyst) to the 'most sweepingly radical critique' (a Canadian) (Wallerstein 1993: 166).

The renowned American analyst Kernberg (1986) is one of several who have described psychoanalytic training as 'all too often conducted in an atmosphere of indoctrination rather than of open scientific exploration' (p. 799). He compares psychoanalytic institutes to 'monasteries or religious retreats and psychoanalysis [to] a system of religious beliefs' (p. 809). In a later article, delightfully titled 'Thirty methods to destroy the creativity of psychoanalytic candidates' (Kernberg 1996), he refers to thirty problems in psychoanalytic education that require attention, including slowing down of the progression of candidates, repetitive and unquestioning teaching of Freud, monolithic tendencies regarding theoretical approaches, the isolation of candidates, discouragement of original contributions by candidates, the intellectual isolation of institutes, lack of full presentation of clinical work by senior members and the neglect of studies of controversies regarding psychoanalytic technique. Despite its apparent conservatism, there are some healthy signs in psychoanalysis of reviewing training, although political manoeuvrings between rival societies in Britain seem to serve to deepen convictions about length rather than breadth of training. Criticisms have also come from the humanistic side, as for example the striking article by Mahrer (1998), which calls attention to such concerns as the identity of psychotherapy, the ownership of psychotherapy, the intellectual content of psychotherapy and the lack of any kind of testing of competence in psychotherapy.

There are nonetheless signs of hope, and here we refer not just to psychoanalysis but to the problems of narrowness in other schools as well. In Britain, three things have woken people up to a new alertness in these matters. The UK Council for Psychotherapy has brought the different training institutes much closer to each other, forcing them to look at what they are doing in a much more critical way, particularly the inspection of one institute by two others that brings to the surface imperfections which have been taken for granted. Although such inspections are limited to the observers coming from the same sections (would that there was an inspector from another section altogether!), there has been recognition of the need to be aware of other forms of therapy. Unfortunately, the same thing has not happened in the field of counselling, and some of the counselling courses are much too narrow, often just offering Rogers or Egan as the answer to everything. Insistence on a core model for the accreditation of a counselling course, as does the British Association for Counselling and Psychotherapy, pushes all but the most resolutely integrative courses in that direction.

Secondly, many courses have been upgraded to masters degree standard through linking with a university. Training institutes have then to conform to standards laid down elsewhere: to clarify aims, specify outcomes, produce up-to-date booklists, pay more attention to the needs of students, and so on. Of course, therapy is only partly an academic subject, and academia has a hard time accepting the idea that a disciplined subjectivity is just as important as any kind of objectivity, even though it is harder to specify and measure.

The third influence is less obviously positive, the invasion of the therapy field by accountants. In the USA, the Managed Care programme puts the funding of therapy into the hands of insurance companies and the like; in Britain, this mostly takes the form of an insistence by funding bodies in the National Health Service and elsewhere that there is empirical validation of 'treatments', particularly through the use of randomized trials of the type used in medicine. At first this only suited certain types of therapy, those with specific short-term aims, although more and more evidence is emerging for this kind of efficacy in a variety of therapeutic approaches. Short-term work tends to limit therapists to the instrumental level, even if they often see the client as a whole person with wider, deeper needs.

Yet one of the most curious things about training is the research showing that untrained people can do just as good a job as trained ones. For example, Hattie *et al.* (1984) identified forty-three pieces of research in which professionals and paraprofessionals were compared in their effectiveness when treating patients. The conclusion was that the paraprofessionals were actually more effective than the professionals. A later critique of this paper by Berman and Norton (1985) went over the data afresh, and found that there was actually no difference between the performance of the two groups.

Russell also surveyed the research literature very thoroughly. Her six main conclusions were (Russell 1981: 6–7):

1 Comparative studies show that the outcome of psychotherapy does not depend upon the school to which the therapist adheres.

2 Experienced therapists are generally more effective than inexperienced therapists, and experienced therapists resemble each other to a greater extent than they resemble less experienced therapists trained in their respective disciplines.
3 Paraprofessionals consistently achieve outcome equal to, or better than, professional outcomes.
4 A professional training analysis does not appear to increase the effectiveness of the therapist.
5 Therapists who have undergone traditional training are no more effective than those who have not, but microcounselling and skills training appear to be useful procedures in the training of therapists.
6 Congruent matching of therapist and patient increases the effectiveness of therapy.

This survey was later updated (Russell 1993) to take account of more recent research, but the basic results did not change.

These are striking findings, but the reason for them may be quite simple. Of all the influences making for success in therapy, the greatest is the readiness of the client for change. Bohart and Tallman (1998) have shown that the client is highly active in the process of therapy, and that most of what happens depends on the activity of the client rather than the activity of the therapist. 'We further argue that all therapy is ultimately self-help and that it is the client who is the therapist' (Bohart and Tallman 1998: 9). For all our concentration on the way in which therapists use themselves, perhaps it is the openness of the therapist to the client's movement towards change that is paramount. Does it then matter what the training of the designated professional is? (See also the forthcoming volume in this series, on *Aims and Outcomes*, by Syme and Elton Wilson.)

Why do we need training? Perhaps one of the main reasons is to help us to deal with unwanted assumptions and false beliefs, so that the main work of training is *unlearning* them. This is very largely a psychological rather than an intellectual task, and in this the processes of personal therapy and supervision are essential. There are nonetheless intellectual assumptions that training and supervision should be challenging, such as the relationship between the internal and the external worlds; between the expertise of the therapist and the expertise of the client; between the individual, the group and society; between cultures; between the objective, the subjective and the intersubjective; between memory and experience; between models of the person, based on such differences as fulfilment and conflict, optimism and pessimism about human nature; between the origins of disturbance and the maintenance of disturbance, the influence of past and present on a person's future; between the cognitive and the emotional; between free will and determinism; between the material (including the physical) and the spiritual.

When we put such a list together, there certainly seems some point in training. It is not so much about accumulation of information, but rather of discarding unwanted assumptions and beliefs, although such a process often means acquiring knowledge before it can be questioned. But perhaps it is neither ultimately about knowledge, nor the questioning of knowledge, as about gaining in wisdom. And wisdom seems a fine objective for the therapist's use of self.

CHAPTER 6

A dialogue: the authors discuss the therapist's use of self

J.R. First, I would like to say that I have learned a tremendous amount from the collaboration with Michael on writing this book. It has been a revelation to see the amount of work that has been done in the analytic field on things like countertransference and projective identification, and by all sorts of people on the wounded healer. I have also learned some new things about self-disclosure.

But for me the most striking thing about this book is its structure. The way this came about may be of interest. In the beginning we talked rather hopefully about doing justice to four schools of therapy – the psychodynamic group, the humanistic group, the cognitive-behavioural group and the systemic group. A lot of the early material was laid out in this way. But one day I was looking at it and checking it over, and it all took a hop, skip and a jump and re-arranged itself quite differently. I suddenly saw that instead of treating the old ground of schools and their differences, which has been done many times in various ways, it would be more exciting to do something else. I had written before in *Counselling* (as it was then) about two ways of doing therapy, which I then called Adjustment and Liberation (Rowan 2000). And since then I have been writing more (Rowan 2001b) about the transpersonal approach to doing therapy. What happened was that these ideas all came together in a rush, so that I saw that this book could have a three-fold structure. In doing so, the names changed a bit and are now I think much more accurate.

The three-fold division comes originally from the work of Ken Wilber (2000). I saw the charts from this book some years before the book itself came out, and was very much influenced by them in my whole view of the world. They are, of course, just an elaboration of the much earlier book *The Atman Project* (Wilber 1980a), which I came across in 1982. His map, based on a great deal of research and experience, says that there are a number of stages in psychospiritual development and that they are quite recognizable to the discerning eye. Of these, three of the most important are: the Mental Ego (the stage at which most of us operate most of the time), the Centaur (a sort of intermediate stage between the personal and the transpersonal, taking on the characteristics of both, as I have described more fully elsewhere (Rowan 2001a)) and the Psychic/Subtle (the first truly transpersonal stage of development).

I suddenly saw that these corresponded with three approaches to therapy: the instrumental, where the emphasis is all on getting it right; the authentic, where the emphasis is on being real; and the transpersonal, where the emphasis is on surrender to something larger. It strikes me now how curious it is that although the largest number of people live, think and work in the first way, most of the theorists and thinkers seem to think and work in the second way. The third way is smaller again, both in theory and practice, I believe. And so it is in this book that Chapter 3, which deals with the second way, is much the longest.

What was also curious, at least to me, is that the psychodynamic theorists, who are often thought by others to be rather rigid and hidebound, came through in that chapter as having a great deal to say about the authentic and spontaneous.

M.J. As you have learned from the psychoanalytic/psychodynamic, I have also learned from the humanistic, in particular the transpersonal. My fear is that we may have done less than justice to the cognitive-behavioural schools, because our subject does not appear to be of particular interest to therapists of that persuasion. But we have to allow for the fact that if we have had some of our opinions changed of each other, we may both have had this happen to us had we similarly been exposed to a cognitive-behavioural therapist with similar views to our own.

I use the term 'views', but I am not sure it is the right word, because it is the way in which a person thinks, feels and reacts to others that I have in mind here. At the risk of caricaturing, which we have studiously tried to avoid, it does appear that there are some rather rigid thinkers, in all schools of therapy, who can only see their own way as the right one. I wonder whether that is something to do with particular personal characteristics. It is a way of being I have myself known, and written about in a book to which we have both contributed (Spinelli and Marshall 2001), where I can see that in the early stages of my enthusiasm for psychoanalytic ideas, I was pretty intolerant of other theories, even if I often kept tactfully quiet and tried to argue my position logically, to convince others through 'right thinking', rather than by being evangelistic. Interestingly, that seemed to me to be an authentic position at the time, although looking back I was surely more in an 'instrumental mode' where the *ideas* dominated me. I am sure that my 'self' as a therapist has changed, and I am not unusual in that.

That is why I liked your suggestion that we revise our original ground-plan, although I think it was not quite as rigidly divided into schools as you remember. So we have looked at three ways of being, the instrumental, authentic and transpersonal. I am unhappy, although as we said in the Introduction I know others think differently, about thinking of these as *levels*; as though we ought to progress from one to the other in our developments as therapists. I can see a clear place for all three ways of being, probably in every session, in adaptation to where we are with a particular client at a particular time. Therapists are like Winnicott's idea of the adaptive mother, reading the signs in her child, and meeting him or her where he or she is; while as the same time recognizing the points at which changes in relating and being are taking place, and allowing these to happen, before meeting the child again in the new position. So the adaptive mother does not lead, nor does she simply mirror, but interacts, making it difficult to know sometimes whether mother (or, indeed, father) is responding to the child, or the child to the parent. That is where the intersubjective has also come into our writing.

I suppose that the necessary rivalry between any two people meant that I was not going to be put in the shade by some of the humanistic and transpersonal writers you cited. I wanted to show how psychoanalytic/psychodynamic thinking and practice could be understood and seen similarly. I did not fabricate this in any way, although I am aware that I was delighted when, in my researches, I found evidence that showed similar ways of being – which, on the whole, matched my own sense of what it is to be a therapist. Perhaps one of the reasons why you were surprised is that much of what I have gleaned comes from American authors; or at least much less from British analysts. That is not to say that there is not some very fine, radical writing also in British psychoanalysis, but when it comes to the politics of therapy, I am afraid I do not wish to be associated with what appear to me to be the expressions of rivalry and defensiveness of territory that hide behind the banners of 'standards'.

But let me raise the one hesitation I have experienced in working with this material, which is not the instrumental (although I have been anxious not to stress the apparently negative side of manualization, and prefer to refer to the value of learning and implementing workable and helpful techniques); neither is it the authentic, which I believe has been the particular movement that has taken place in my own development as a therapist, partly because of the need to be able to be 'me', partly also under the influence of Peter Lomas (1981), whose work I have admired and whose friendship I have valued.

The less comfortable area is the transpersonal. This may appear strange, given my original training was for the church, where prayer and meditation was the thing! One of the difficulties I have with the transpersonal is that the language implies a more definitive concept than I am happy with – and that may be the case with some of our readers too. I will not go into that here at any length, because I have written about what seem to me to be two ways of approaching 'that which lies beyond', if I can put it that way (Jacobs 2000a: ch. 6). One way is very much expressed in terms that are similar to or identical with spirituality in religion; the other is to express the 'beyond' in elusive, often contradictory terms, indicating that there may be something more and that in all probability there is something more, but we have not got any idea what 'it' is. It is, if you like, agnosticism rather than gnosticism, using both these terms in a positive way, not as suggesting negative or nihilistic thinking in relation to agnosticism, nor inflated enlightenment in relation to gnosticism.

While I therefore easily identify with the instrumental and the authentic – although at the same time remain unsure whether we can ever define 'authentic' or 'real' any more (as we said in Chapter 1) than we can define 'self' – I do not know whether I really engage in a transpersonal way as a therapist, or if I do whether it is in my case much different from being authentic. In other words, I am content as a therapist to be 'taken over' by the session, and the material, and the feelings that pass between myself and the client, or are solely in me. I am content to remain in a state of 'nothingness', not searching for answers, ideas or even for intuition. So what may happen is that I am then 'struck' by an idea, which I may choose to express, and the feeling of being struck comes from I know not where – Jove's thunderbolt perhaps! But is this my transpersonal self, or my authentic self?

J.R. I like what you say, and would like to embroider a bit on two points you make. The first one is about the instrumental approach. I agree entirely when you say that it is very important and not to be downgraded or treated as of lesser importance. In fact, it is my suspicion that most therapists, most of the time, work in this way, whatever their espoused theory. In other words, we continually drop into treating the client or patient like an object, and it is inevitable that we should do so. Our whole culture is constructed in this way, where we are systematically rewarded for playing roles instead of being fully human. And every time we play a role as therapists, we are occupying the instrumental space rather than the authentic or the transpersonal space.

It would be a fault, in my view, if a therapist felt guilty every time he or she became instrumental. In my experience, the worst form of therapy from this point of view is the person-centred position. People from this school continually speak as if they should be authentic at all times, and should feel guilty if they fail to be so. But some of the comments in the book by Farber and his associates (1996) make it clear that even Carl Rogers did not follow his own precepts at all times. Perhaps those of us who follow in his footsteps do not need to be more perfect than him. Perhaps we can admit to the truth and forgive ourselves as necessary. Similar remarks apply to psychodramatists, some of whom seem to want to be spontaneous and creative at all times.

The other point I would like to take up is the question as to what frame of mind we are in at any given moment in our work as therapists. The example you give, of surrendering to the moment and waiting to be struck by something, seems clearly transpersonal to me. But this does not mean that it is not authentic. It is just that it does mean going beyond *just* being authentic. The authentic position, as we are describing it here, insists on ownership. I own and take responsibility for all my actions. They come from me, they belong to me. If I am creative, it is me being creative. As soon as we go beyond this, and open ourselves up to the possibility of something just coming to us from we know not where, we are going beyond that and into the realm of the transpersonal.

I think you are right to indicate that the transpersonal is more tricky to handle than the other two positions. This is simply because, I suggest, our culture is so uneducated about spirituality and so lacking in a language in which to talk about it. There are to my mind five definitions of spirituality. The most popular is that spirituality involves peak experiences or altered states, which can be reached also, sometimes perhaps, through the appropriate use of drugs. The second is that it involves the highest levels in any seriously pursued realm of development, such as science, art, philosophy or sport – a philosophical definition, which is also quite widespread and widely studied. Thirdly, that spirituality is a separate developmental line itself, pursued through meditation, prayer, ritual, contemplation, and so forth. This is the most popular definition among religious people, who often want to say that their approach is the only true one, although Paul Tillich has shown that we can talk about *ultimate concern* in a meaningful but non-exclusive way. On this definition we can say that there can be prepersonal, personal and transpersonal forms of spirituality. The fourth definition is similar, that spirituality is the sum total of the highest levels of all the developmental lines, which implies that nothing would count as spirituality unless it were fully and completely transpersonal. The fifth definition is that it is an attitude (such as openness, trust or love) that we may or may not have at any stage: the broadest but vaguest (see Wilber 1983, 2000).

I myself lean towards the third definition, although I prefer the word 'transpersonal' to 'spiritual'. Does any of this throw light on your reservations?

M.J. This makes sense, but at the same time illustrates for me the difficulty with the term 'transpersonal' – although I am anxious not to get into a debate about that here, unless it is relevant to the therapist's use of self. Words like 'spiritual', and terms like 'soul' and even the word 'mind', often presume the existence of something that is not readily identifiable or accessible to critical analysis, and yet to which is attached such significance that it tends to become 'greater' than anything else. 'Transpersonal' in many of your definitions appears to mean something 'above' the usual, like the second one, which is my preference in that list, because it does not confine the 'pursuit' to the spiritual. But some of the other definitions (the fifth is an exception) imply an 'aboveness', which smacks of metaphysics. The Freudian streak in me is suspicious of such talk.

But as I think about it, and consult the dictionary to look at other words with the prefix 'trans-', and return more obviously to our theme of the therapist's use of self, I want to extend my mental picture of transpersonal, so that (for me at least) it means 'across' and 'through' as in the words 'transatlantic' or 'transparent', rather than 'above'. Despite what we have said about levels in Chapter 1, I am concerned at how the word is generally understood and can be used to mean 'superior', implying then that all else is 'inferior'. Then I begin to wonder whether what we are therefore describing in our three positions is something like this:

- *The instrumental*. The therapist engages with the client through techniques (sometimes even going as far as what we have called manualization), and completely attends to the client, setting aside self-interest, but also self-reflection and the use of self as we have described it in the second position.
- *The authentic*. The therapist meets with and engages with the client additionally through attending to and experiencing what is going on within the therapist, through self-reflection, and monitoring her or his own feelings and thoughts. These may be understood sometimes as coming from the influence of the client's presence, consciously and unconsciously conveying messages to the therapist, or from the client's material. This is one psychoanalytic view, of countertransference as the response to the patient's transference; but which may also be to do with what the therapist experiences apparently independently of the client, yet still potentially relevant to that piece of therapeutic work.
- *The transpersonal*. The therapist engages with what is passing *between or beyond* the therapist and client, in one way not attending to anything, neither self nor the client; but still open to feelings, thoughts and experiences that appear to come from nowhere. The therapist needs to attend to these experiences, and this (attending to those perceptions, intuitive flashes, etc.) seems to me to mean returning to the authentic position, and working on what is going on within oneself. This will hopefully suggest whether the experience of an idea or a feeling or an image 'breaking in' to oneself is valid or not (authentic or not). Then the therapist needs the help of the instrumental position to decide how best to express what he or she has experienced, in such a way as it can serve the primary concern, the interest of the client, rather than becoming an 'ego-trip' for the therapist. This sounds like a long process, but I suggest that in experienced therapists this process can take as long as a dream – that is, a few seconds.

I have a second response to what you write about definitions of transpersonal, which goes a little beyond our theme, but comes out of the process of writing, and our own discovery of common areas of concern, going sometimes under different labels. I am made more aware just how artificial are the words that are used to distinguish different orientations; if 'transpersonal' includes 'across' and 'through' the personal as well as 'beyond', it becomes a term that most therapists of whatever orientation could subscribe to – and then, perhaps, pay more attention to. Similarly, 'person-centred' really cannot be claimed by one orientation, inasmuch as all therapies are concerned for the person who is the client, even if the different therapies employ various techniques to serve that concern. There is no reason why functioning at what we have called the instrumental level need be any the less person-centred. In the paragraph above, I describe how in my view the therapist needs to flow between the levels, translating any 'transpersonal' experience into a 'person-centred' concern – that is, how to convey this in a way that has real meaning for the client. Gestalt, and its emphasis on the whole, is what we are trying to arrive at as we discuss the constituent elements of the therapist's use of self. And the psychodynamic, as well as the analysis of the dynamic, is present not simply in the relationship between therapist and client, and within the therapist and the client's unique inner worlds and histories, but in the dynamic interplay between instrumental, authentic and transpersonal, such as I have described immediately above.

J.R. I don't think that we are going to arrive at a neat foolproof definition of the transpersonal, and I am not at all sure that we need or want to. In any case, being in the public domain, it is being redefined all the time through its use by various parties. All I would urge is that anyone who uses the word take due account of the existing literature, and particularly of the great pioneers such as Jung, Assagioli, Maslow, Grof and Wilber. To write about the transpersonal without paying due attention to these groundbreaking figures seems folly to me.

I have read several books recently (Wellings and McCormick 2000; Young-Eisendrath and Miller 2000; King-Spooner and Newnes 2001) that have made this mistake, plus the mistake of confusing spirituality with religion. They also make the important mistake, which Wilber (1980b) identified over twenty years ago and labelled the 'pre/trans fallacy', of confusing what is prepersonal and what is transpersonal. But I recognize that it is easy to run into all sorts of errors in relation to the transpersonal, largely because it is unfamiliar territory in our culture. In spite of your doubts, I think we have been clear enough in our Chapters 4 and 5 to obviate most of the likely misunderstandings.

Enough said about defining the transpersonal! Another area interests me a good deal. Before we began, I found it hard to see how a psychoanalyst could be authentic. It seemed obvious to me that such people hid behind a role that made them quite impervious to any access by the client. But I have now come across enough exceptions to see that it is indeed possible. One cannot read Searles, for example, without realizing that his authenticity consists not only in his being in touch with his conscious reactions to clients, but also in his being ready to engage in a genuine dialogue with the client based on his awareness of his own countertransference. This ability was, I think, hard won through his own work on himself. And having found one such shining example, I then started to find more. I am sure you had a different starting point, but did anything like this happen to you too?

M.J. To address your question, I need to comment on the word 'authentic', just as I needed to unpack the term 'transpersonal'. What 'authentic' may appear to mean (at least in the discourse of therapy) is that style of being a therapist which involves openness to the 'real' self, which, in turn, probably means self-disclosure and even being more active. But 'authentic' can also mean 'true to one self' and, if we recognize, as we surely must, that psychoanalysts are trying to be as true to themselves as much as any other therapist, is there any reason why the relatively silent analyst should be any the less authentic than the more expressive person-centred therapist – just to take stereotypical extremes? If my training, as any type of therapist, suggests that I need to behave in a certain way, and if that way suits my personality, so that the training fits me like a glove, then it is unlikely that I am simply adopting a role. There is a match between the therapeutic style I have chosen to be trained in and my own personality. It seems to me difficult, then, to say that such therapists are not being authentic, whatever their form of practice. Whether being authentic in that sense is enough is a different question.

I happen to agree with you that people like Searles, Winnicott and Lomas are obviously very much in touch with themselves, and in Lomas' (1973) case that is made even more obvious to his patients than I think even by Searles (1965) or by Winnicott – see Guntrip (1975, 1996) and Little (1990) for Winnicott's openness. Another example would be the existential therapist Yalom (1989; Yalom and

Elkin 1974), whose case studies show an obvious authenticity, as you and I have been using the word. But if Lomas or Yalom make being real more obvious by what they sometimes share with a patient, authenticity also comes from the way a person *is* as much as the way they *act* or *speak*. So is not the more blank-screen, passive analyst also authentic, true to himself or herself, not only because he or she believes a particular style, and stays true to that belief, but also because it suits that person's own way of being? He or she is not adopting a role. It is interesting that I find it impossible immediately to think of an actual example, and this may be because the type of person I am now describing is unlikely to 'go public', both because it is not in their nature and they do not think it right to discuss practice in print. It is the very advertising of their approach that reinforces our perception of Searles and others as authentic. But have we any evidence to suggest that others, who say less, are less authentic?

But, of course, if any therapist were acting a part that is not 'them', then it would appear that he or she is not authentic, and is simply acting in an instrumental way. That criticism could certainly apply to those who train as analysts, and 'adopt' the analytic stance, without matching their personality; although it is possible to envisage a somewhat defensively garrulous trainee as not only learning to be more silent with patients, but also becoming more relaxed as the result of personal therapy, and being less garrulous in other settings too. Learning to be a more effective therapist may also deepen other relationships in other settings. In the same way, thinking about the inauthentic, what I say could apply equally to the humanistic therapist who to the casual observer looks as if he or she is being authentic, but in fact is putting it on, adopting the role of what they think their sort of therapist should be like. I can think of people I have seen in practice sessions, apparently being empathic and genuine, but where you feel it is just an act.

This has bearing on my answer to your question about what happened to me in my training. I should point out that I am not an analyst, and that I do not even call myself a psychoanalytic psychotherapist, even though my training has largely been in psychoanalysis. My label of 'psychodynamic' is intended to advertise a broader approach to therapy. At first I think my training in psychoanalytic technique suited me. I was being authentic at the time, inasmuch as in the beginning, when I was very uncertain about how much I really knew and perhaps about what on earth I was doing, the more silent, passive, interpretative approach suited me – it fitted, if not quite like a glove. I was also genuinely matching my state of mind as a therapist with my behaviour as a therapist (for a fuller description, see Jacobs 2001). At that time I valued the 'blank-screen' approach. But as I acquired more confidence, I certainly then began to feel that some of what I was practising no longer felt comfortable, and that I was having to restrict my responses – the methods that I had learned and adopted to that point were not enough. To be more 'me' I needed to be able to be more interactive, without feeling that I was being an intrusive therapist by saying rather more. I needed to be more disclosing, without thinking it was an error of technique. As I have grown in experience I have trusted the intuitive more (the transpersonal as you would perhaps put it), and expressed my hunches more readily (as we might imagine the authentic therapist would). I have been comfortable with not being an expert, but at the same time have actually felt a much greater sense of my expertise. So, to remain true to myself, my way of being as a therapist changed as I changed, just as much as being a therapist changed me.

There are certain times in life when we radically question what we have learned. Some people at such times might adopt a different therapeutic approach – many certainly become more integrative. But it also happens (at least it has to me with regard to psychoanalysis) that we realize that what we have learned has been one-sided, and that there are other ways of being a therapist, which in my case some other analysts clearly demonstrate. Perhaps it is then that we discover Searles, Winnicott, Lomas, etc. – when we are ready for them. But a stage further on I think we also discover that our views of those we thought were much more 'traditional' (like Freud) are also one-sided. If we take Searles as an example, he recounts how when he first experienced his Oedipal countertransference, his training told him that he was not yet sufficiently analysed. But he explored this more, including through private conversations with other analysts about what they actually experienced rather than what they said in public that they experienced. He was able to recognize that what was happening to him was saying more about a particular stage of the therapeutic relationship, and that he could use his feelings as indications of what was happening to his relationship to his patients, and theirs to him (Searles 1959: 284–5). It may therefore sometimes (even often) be that in the questioning of what we have learned, we have to start unlearning; and it may also be that in questioning what we have learned, that we learn that we have not yet learned enough of what was already obviously there, but which we were not yet ready to recognize.

I am suggesting, then, that the expression of being authentic may well change, and that the essential thing is for the person we are as a therapist to match the person we are as ourselves (vague terms, I know, but you will know what I mean). But I suspect there is another feature that we need to take into account: that authenticity is the product of the therapeutic relationship and not just the way a therapist is and acts. There are some clients where it is possible to be more authentic, to be more myself, where it feels that many of my responses to them reflect the way I am experiencing them; and there are other clients who make it impossible for me to be authentic, where I have to be more on my guard as to what I can say. Or perhaps that is the wrong way of putting it; rather that with some clients it is authentic for me to be one way, and with other clients it is authentic for me to be another way. And perhaps that depends upon whether they are themselves reaching a point of greater authenticity. Those who present a 'false self', and who are frightened of what may happen when the false self is taken away, are the clients who I suspect need us to be much more circumspect in the way we are with them and in what we say to them; whereas those who have allowed themselves to give up much of the pretence they have had about themselves and others, are the clients where it feels possible to be more 'oneself'.

J.R. Yes, I agree with that. In fact, I once wrote a piece in which I said that the ideal form of therapy, involving total openness, was very rare, simply because the client was not ready for it, even if the therapist was. What you say about development also resonates with me. When I first discovered my own subpersonalities, I found that there was one named Brown Cow who took over when I acted as a therapist. Brown Cow was very warm and accepting, very accurate in perception and was very good at leading groups. Later she merged with another character to become Jean Starry, a French existential androgyne, who also wrote book reviews. But both of those faded out when I became more authentic.

I have rather a strict analysis of what is meant by authentic, which I have written about elsewhere (Rowan 2001a: 42–4). For me, as for Wilber (2000: 197–217), it represents a definite stage in psychospiritual development, with the emergence of an existential consciousness, or what Maslow calls self-actualization. We talked about this rather precisely in Chapter 1. If I had to choose just one quotation to sum it up, it would have to be the one from Bugental:

By authenticity I mean a central genuineness and awareness of being. Authenticity is that presence of an individual in his living in which he is fully aware in the present moment, in the present situation. Authenticity is difficult to convey in words, but experientially it is readily perceived in ourselves or in others. Authenticity has three functional characteristics: 1. The authentic person is broadly aware of himself, his relationships, and his world in all dimensions. 2. The authentic person accepts and seems to go to meet the fact that he is constantly in the process of making choices, that decisions are the very stuff of living. 3. The authentic person takes responsibility for his decisions, including full recognition of their consequences. It is here that the terrible threat of authenticity resides.

(Bugental 1981: 102–3)

Going back now to your examples, I think it is right to say that when we are with an inauthentic person it may be quite appropriate to be inauthentic ourselves. Or, to put it in the terms we have been using in this book, if we are with a client who is clearly only looking for an instrumental solution, it may be quite appropriate to adopt an instrumental attitude ourselves. This is called being flexible. There is nothing wrong with being authentic and being flexible. In fact, it reminds me of the stirring words of Bergantino (1981: 53): 'Being tricky and authentic can be two sides of the same coin. Being an authentic trickster will not destroy the patient's confidence if the therapist's heart is in the right place'.

But if Wilber is right, the limits assert themselves if someone at one level tries to operate at another level without having been through the change in consciousness required to operate at that level. Your example of the people who in practice sessions seem to be putting on an act might be an instance of this. They could be people who have not yet reached the level in their own psycho-spiritual development of the authentic (the integrated, the existential, the actualized, etc.) and are still stuck at the instrumental level (mental ego, consensus trance, conformist, inauthentic, etc.). They are then acting as if they were authentic, as best they can, and producing what Mearns has called a portrayal. The demands of a training course can easily evoke this kind of thing, and there is no escape from it other than the personal development of the trainee involved.

I would say that there is no form of therapy that does not raise these sorts of issues. I once went to an event where there were five therapists on the platform, all from different schools. And one of them, speaking of the behaviourist who had most sternly abjured any mention of human warmth or contact, said: 'I work just down the corridor from him, and I can assure you that when he welcomes a client into his office, he displays massive quantities of unconditional positive regard!' The idea that therapists always behave as the textbooks might lead us to expect seems just false to me.

Even with all that said, however, it is hard for me to see how the unreconstructed analyst you describe, who sits silent behind the head of the patient, and never utters a word other than interpretations, could be anything other than instrumental. When you write 'because he or she believes a particular style, and stays true to that belief', that seems to me the epitome of the instrumental approach. So it actually seems to me that saying that someone is psychodynamic hardly tells us more than saying that someone is eclectic. We would have to see the person in action with a range of different clients before we could have any idea of where he or she fitted in our scheme.

I think what we are about – what the whole book is really about – is helping people to be more aware of what they are doing, so that they are not kidding themselves, and not kidding anyone else, about what they are doing and where they stand.

M.J. I did not use the term 'unreconstructed', so your addition may in fact prevent you understanding the point I am making. I am assuming the analyst has had their own therapy, and that the person matches the style; and that even if the style is one of being silent, and offering few, but effective, interpretations, that is as much being authentic as sharing personal feelings evoked by the therapeutic relationship. And at this point an example *does* come to mind, one that fits what I was writing about those who have chosen not to advertise their style. The example comes from Guntrip's (1996: 739–54 reproduced from 1975: 145–56) account of his analysis with W.R.D. Fairbairn, the Scottish analyst who was somewhat independent of the Freud/Klein debates in London, and whose writing is mainly about the structure of the personality – a theoretical though quite radical view. Guntrip had his first analysis with Fairbairn in the 1950s and then went on to see Winnicott for a second analysis. He clearly got different things from each, and the breakthrough to his amnesia concerning a life-long trauma came when he was no longer seeing either, through a dream the night after he had heard of Winnicott's death.

It is Fairbairn who provides the interesting example here. He once said to Guntrip: 'You can go on analysing for ever and get no-where. It's the personal relation that is therapeutic. Science has no values except scientific values, the schizoid values of the investigator who stands outside of life and watches. It is purely instrumental, useful for a time but then you have to get back to living' (Guntrip 1996: 741). You will have noted the word 'instrumental', which is pertinent here. But Guntrip describes how, although this was Fairbairn's stated view

> of the 'mirror analyst', a non-relating observer simply inter-preting . . . in spite of his conviction Fairbairn did not have the same capacity for natural, spontaneous 'personal relating' that Winnicott had. With me he was more of a 'technical interpreter' than he thought he was, or than I expected . . . In general I found Fairbairn becoming more orthodox in practice than in theory while Winnicott was more revolutionary in practice than in theory.
>
> (Guntrip 1996: 741–2)

The paper deserves more complete attention than I can give it here, as Guntrip describes Fairbairn's consulting room, and the seat-ing arrangements, the 'slightly formal air', 'odd for an analyst who did not believe in the "mirror-analyst" theory' (Guntrip 1996: 744). But it is interesting that if he was formal in sessions, the two men met after the sessions and 'discussed theory and he would unbend, and I found the human Fairbairn as we talked face to face. Realistic-ally, he was my understanding good father after sessions, and in sessions in the transference he was my dominating bad mother imposing exact interpretations' (Guntrip 1996: 742). And when they parted for the last time 'I suddenly realised that in all that long period we had never once shaken hands, and he was letting me leave without that friendly gesture. I put out my hand and at once he took it, and I suddenly saw a few tears trickle down his face. *I saw the warm heart of this man with a fine mind and a shy nature*' (Guntrip 1996: 745, emphasis in original).

Now this account raises all manner of questions about authenti-city and instrumentality. Guntrip is critical of his analysis with Fairbairn – he could not accept the constant stream of Oedipal interpretations, although through his negative response he really understood how dominating his own mother was. Guntrip's theoret-ical work is much influenced by Fairbairn's model of personality structure, indicating the other side, the positive transference. He appears to have gained much from the analysis, and when he went on to see Winnicott he gained a different perspective, enabling Guntrip to find 'an ultimate good mother' (Guntrip 1996: 749). But the healing came after both men were dead. So if we are asking what makes for effective therapy (and that is the point of Guntrip's article), we might say that both analysts helped, the instrumental and the authentic, but in the end it was a dream (the transpersonal) that enabled the ultimate shift to take place.

We have, of course, not denied the value of the instrumental; but I think the point I am making about Fairbairn is that that was for him the only authentic way he could be, even if he could unbend in the post-session discussions. It is remarkable for me to find Guntrip using a very similar phrase to my own earlier in relation to this question. He writes of Fairbairn: 'The unpredictable factor of "natural fit" enters in' (Guntrip 1996: 741). My sense is that Fairbairn did not adopt that style as an analyst, but that he was being truly Fairbairn. Guntrip also acknowledges his own part in creating the formality. But I have no reason to doubt Fairbairn's genuineness.

I was speaking recently with a music therapist about playing his working method and about the instruments he encourages his young patients to play. I commented on the difference I had perceived at an orchestral concert between a young extremely virtuoso violinist's technique, which was superb, and her interpretation of the music, which had seemed to me to lack 'soul'. The music therapist commented that, in using instruments with his clients, he is not concerned about their technical ability, because he is providing an opportunity for them to use the instrument to express themselves – often their anguish or isolation. When it comes to therapists, I would like to see them use their instruments well, whether it is a questionnaire or skills of listening and responding. But I also want to know that their 'soul' is in the work too. I have no way of being able to prove it, but reading Guntrip's article, I have no doubt that Fairbairn's soul was there, and that his silent, interpretive stance was not the mark of the purely instrumental, but an indication of the authentic 'shy nature' of the man.

I wonder what this has to say about the development of the concept of the therapist's use of self?

J.R. It seems to me that you are fighting against any real separation between the instrumental and the authentic forms of consciousness. Yet if we look at the research referred to in Chapter 1, there is a wide gap between the instrumental and the authentic, such that most people live and work at the instrumental level and have little or no authentic awareness. I believe this is true of therapists as well. And the reason for this is fear. To be authentic is to be open and vulnerable. Most people do not want to be vulnerable. And this fear can be rationalized. It seems to me that many therapists are not aiming at liberation, and that they may indeed regard it as something dangerous:

> Indeed, it is clear to me that society needs men to have unresolved Oedipus complexes; that we continue to live with the fear of the father (the Law). A truly free man would represent a real threat to social organization.
>
> (Jukes 1993: 114)

There is a fear here, a fear of social disorganization. If the boundaries of control were broken, all kinds of bad things might happen. The fear in the therapist is of disorganization of the self, or of the client, or of the relationship between them; and catastrophic expectations on the part of the therapist that make them restrict their work to what is safe and unexceptional. One of the favourite slogans at the instrumental stage is: 'We don't pretend to know better than the client. We let the client set the agenda and the aims'. This assumes, of course, that there is just one type of client, the rational one who makes a clear contract.

But perhaps it is sometimes the irrational one, the neurotic one, who makes the contract with us, with the rational one nowhere to be seen? This sort of suggestion is often resisted at this stage by the instrumental therapist with robust common sense, saying things like:

> When the going got tough [in restricting his rituals], George typically suggested that it might be better for us to explore the meaning behind his symptoms. I would react, using my 'tough army sergeant stance' by pointing out that he had devoted six years of his life to exploring meanings and dynamics to no avail.
>
> (Lazarus 1989: 234)

There are many ways of avoiding authenticity, and this is just one of them. The way I read your account, Fairbairn clearly had his own method too.

But lest it be thought that we are saying that cognitive-behavioural therapists are automatically instrumental, meaning not authentic, Dryden (1991) records that he had sent one client a birthday card: 'I want to stress that I did not see this purely as a technique. If I did not experience the concern, I would not have given him the card' (p. 141). It is obviously possible for cognitive-behavioural therapists to be authentic: it is a choice that many of them and therapists of other persuasions make, to restrict themselves to the instrumental.

There is, of course, no such thing as an ideal therapist. What the main thrust of this book has shown is that there are different expressions of the therapist's use of self, and I hope that what we have done is to open up this subject to further debate, research and exploration. We have argued that there is a difference between the instrumental therapist, the authentic therapist and the transpersonal therapist, a greater difference perhaps than between orientations. They have different aims, different beliefs and different notions of the self. But I think it is harder to be an authentic therapist than it is to be an instrumental therapist, and harder to be a transpersonal therapist than it is to be an authentic one. It seems to me that some therapists are going to find some of what we have written as deeply unacceptable, simply because it offers them a kind of mirror in which they may see themselves. And do they like what they see?

References

Aponte, H.J. and Winter, J.E. (2000) The person and practice of the therapist: treatment and training, in M. Baldwin (ed.) *The Use of Self in Therapy*, 2nd edn. New York: Haworth Press.

Aponte, J.F. and Lyons, M.J. (1980) Supervision in community settings: concepts, methods and issues, in A.K. Hess (ed.) *Psychotherapy Supervision: Theory, Research and Practice*. New York: Wiley.

Aron, L. (1991) The patient's experience of the analyst's subjectivity, *Psychoanalytic Dialogues*, 1: 29–51.

Bacal, H. (1985) Optimal responsiveness and the therapeutic process, in A. Goldberg (ed.) *Progress in Self Psychology*, Vol. 1. Hillsdale, NJ: Analytic Press.

Baldwin, M. (ed.) (2000) *The Use of Self in Therapy*, 2nd edn. New York: Haworth Press.

Baldwin, P.A. (1997) *Four and Twenty Blackbirds*. Las Vegas, CA: Bramble Books.

Balint, M. (1948) On the psycho-analytic training system, *International Journal of Psycho-analysis*, 29: 163–73.

Balint, M. (1968) *The Basic Fault*. London: Tavistock.

Balint, M. and Balint, A. (1939) On transference and counter-transference, in M. Balint and A. Balint (1965) *Primary Love and Psycho-Analytic Technique*. London: Tavistock.

Barnes, M. and Berke, J. (1973) *Mary Barnes: Two Accounts of a Journey Through Madness*. London: Penguin.

Barron, J.W. and Hoffer, A. (1994) Historical events reinforcing Freud's emphasis on 'holding down the countertransference', *Psychoanalytic Quarterly*, 63: 536–40.

Beebe, J. (1995) Sustaining the potential analyst's morale, in P. Kugler (ed.) *Jungian Perspectives on Clinical Supervision*. Einsiedeln: Daimon.

Beier, E.G. and Young, D.M. (1980) Supervision in communications analytic therapy, in A.K. Hess (ed.) *Psychotherapy Supervision: Theory, Research and Practice*. New York: Wiley.

Belenky, M.F., Clinchy, B.M., Goldberger, N.R. and Tarule, J.M. (1986) *Women's Ways of Knowing: The Development of Self, Voice and Mind*. New York: Basic Books.

Benedek, T. (1969) Training analysis – past, present and future, *International Journal of Psycho-Analysis*, 50: 437–45.

Bergantino, L. (1981) *Psychotherapy, Insight and Style*. Boston, MA: Allyn & Bacon.

Berman, J.S. and Norton, N.C. (1985) Does professional training make a therapist more effective?, *Psychological Bulletin*, 94: 2.

Berne, E. (1961) *Transactional Analysis in Psychotherapy*. New York: Grove Press.

Binswanger, L. (1958a) The existential analysis school of thought, in R. May, E. Angel and H.F. Ellenberger (eds) *Existence: A New Dimension in Psychiatry and Psychology*. New York: Basic Books.

Binswanger, L. (1958b) The case of Ellen West: an anthropological clinical study, in R. May, E. Angel and H.F. Ellenberger (eds) *Existence: A New Dimension in Psychiatry and Psychology*. New York: Basic Books.

Binswanger, L. (1963) *Being in the World*. New York: Basic Books.

Bion, W.R. (1961) *Experience in Groups and Other Papers*. London: Tavistock.

Bion, W.R. (1962) *Learning from Experience*. London: Karnac Books.

Bion, W.R. (1965) *Transformations*. London: Heinemann.

Bion, W.R. (1967) *Second Thoughts*. New York: Jason Aronson/London: Heinemann.

Bion, W.R. (1970) *Attention and Interpretation*. London: Tavistock.

Bion, W.R. (1992) *Cogitations*. London: Karnac Books.

Blatner, A. (1994) Tele, in P. Holmes, M. Karp and M. Watson (eds) *Psychodrama Since Moreno: Innovations in Theory and Practice*. London: Routledge.

Bohart, A.C. and Tallman, K. (1998) The person as active agent in experiential therapy, in L.S. Greenberg, J.C. Watson and G. Lietaer (eds) *Handbook of Experiential Psychotherapy*. New York: Guilford Press.

Bollas, C. (1987) *The Shadow of the Object*. London: Free Association Books.

Boorstein, S. (ed.) (1996) *Transpersonal Psychotherapy*, 2nd edn. Albany, NY: State University of New York Press.

Bragdon, E. (1988) *A Sourcebook for Helping People in Spiritual Emergency*. Los Altos, CA: Lightening Up Press.

Brazier, D. (2001) *Zen Therapy*, 2nd edn. London: Constable Robinson.

Brenner, C. (1976) *Psychoanalytic Technique and Psychic Conflict*. New York: International Universities Press.

Brinich, P. and Shelley, C. (2002) *The Self and Personality Structure*. Buckingham: Open University Press.

Britton, R. (1998) *Belief and Imagination: Explorations in Psychoanalysis*. London: Routledge.

Brookes, C.E. (1995) On supervision in Jungian continuous case seminars, in P. Kugler (ed.) *Jungian Perspectives on Clinical Supervision*. Einsiedeln: Daimon.

Brothers, B.J. (ed.) (2000) *The Personhood of the Therapist*. Binghamton, NY: Haworth Press.

Bruzzone, M., Casaula, E., Jimenez, J.P. and Jordan, J.F. (1985) Regression and persecution in analytic training: reflections on experience, *International Review of Psycho-Analysis*, 12: 411–15.

Buber, M. (1970) *I and Thou* (trans. W. Kaufmann). Edinburgh: T. & T. Clark.

Buber, M. (1985) *Between Man and Man* (trans. R.G. Smith). New York: Macmillan.

Buber, M. (1988) *The Knowledge of Man: A Philosophy of the Interhuman* (trans. M. Friedman and R.G. Smith). Atlantic Highlands: Humanities Press.

Buckley, P. (1997) Review of personal relations therapy: the collected papers of H.J.S. Guntrip, *Journal of the American Psychoanalytic Association*, 45: 581–2.

Budgell, R. (1995) Being touched through space. Unpublished dissertation, School of Psychotherapy and Counselling, Regents College, London.

Bugental, J.F.T. (1978) *Psychotherapy and Process: The Fundamentals of an Existential-Humanistic Approach*. Reading, MA: Addison-Wesley.

Bugental, J.F.T. (1981) *The Search for Authenticity* (enlarged edition). New York: Irvington.

Bugental, J.F.T. and Sterling, M. (1995) Existential-humanistic psychotherapy: new perspectives, in A.S. Gurman and S.B. Messer (eds) *Essential Psychotherapies*. New York: Guilford Press.

Burke, W.F. and Tansey, M.J. (1991) Countertransference disclosure and models of therapeutic action, *Contemporary Psychoanalysis*, 27: 351–84.

Carroll, M. (1996) *Counselling Supervision: Theory, Skills and Practice*. London: Cassell.

Cinnirella, M. and Loewenthal, K.M. (1999) Religious and ethnic group influences on beliefs about mental illness: a qualitative interview study, *British Journal of Medical Psychology*, 72(4): 505–24.

Clarkson, P. (1995) *The Therapeutic Relationship*. London: Whurr.

Clarkson, P. (1998) Supervised supervision: including the archetopoi of supervision, in P. Clarkson (ed.) *Supervision: Psychoanalytic and Jungian Perspectives*. London: Whurr.

Cobb, N. (1997) On the sublime: Eva Loewe and the practice of psychotherapy, or Aphrodite in the consulting room, in P. Clarkson (ed.) *On the Sublime in Psychoanalysis, Archetypal Psychology and Psychotherapy*. London: Whurr.

Cooper, D. (1967) *Psychiatry and Anti-Psychiatry*. London: Tavistock.

Cooper, J. and Seal, P. (2000) Neuro-linguistic programming, in C. Feltham and I. Horton (eds) *Handbook of Counselling and Psychotherapy*. London: Sage.

Corbett, L. (1995) Supervision and the mentor archetype, in P. Kugler (ed.) *Jungian Perspectives on Clinical Supervision*. Einsiedeln: Daimon.

Corbin, H. (1969) *Creative Imagination in the Sufism of Ibn 'Arabi*. Princeton, NJ: Princeton University Press.

Cortright, B. (1997) *Psychotherapy and Spirit*. Albany, NY: State University of New York Press.

Couch, A.S. (1995) Anna Freud's adult psychoanalytic technique: a defence of classical analysis, *International Journal of Psycho-Analysis*, 76: 153–71.

Cowley, A.-D.S. and Adams, R.S. (2000) On Satir's use of self, in B.J. Brothers (ed.) *The Personhood of the Therapist*. Binghamton, NY: Haworth Press.

Daniels, T.G., Rigazio-Digilio, S.A. and Ivey, A.E. (1997) Microcounselling: a training and supervision paradigm for the helping professions, in C.E. Watkins (ed.) *Handbook of Psychotherapy Supervision*. New York: Wiley.

Dass, R. and Gorman, P. (1996) *How Can I Help?* New York: Knopf.

Dineen, T. (1996) *Manufacturing Victims: What the Psychology Industry is Doing to People*. New York: Robert Davis.

Dryden, W. (1991) *Dryden on Counselling, Vol. 1: Seminal Papers*. London: Whurr.

Dryden, W. (ed.) (1993) *Questions and Answers on Counselling in Action*. London: Sage.

Dryden, W. (1995) Rational emotive behaviour therapy, in M. Walker (ed.) *Morag: Myself or Mother-hen?* Buckingham: Open University Press.

Dryden, W. (2000) Rational emotive behaviour therapy, in C. Feltham and I. Horton (eds) *Handbook of Counselling and Psychotherapy*. London: Sage.

Dupont, J. (1995) *The Clinical Diary of Sandor Ferenczi*. Cambridge, MA: Harvard University Press.

Egan, G. (1994) *The Skilled Helper*. Belmont, CA: Brooks/Cole.

Eigen, M. (1998) *The Psychoanalytic Mystic*. London: Free Association Books.

Eisler, R. (1987) *The Chalice and the Blade*. San Francisco, CA: Harper & Row.

Ekstein, R. and Wallerstein, R.S. (1972) *The Teaching and Learning of Psychotherapy* (revised edition). New York: International Universities Press.

Ellis, A. and Yeager, R.J. (1989) *Why Some Therapies Don't Work*. Buffalo, NY: Prometheus Books.

Epstein, M. (1996) *Thoughts Without a Thinker: Psychotherapy from a Buddhist Perspective*. New York: Basic Books.

Erikson, E. (1965) *Childhood and Society*. London: Penguin.

Farber, B.A., Brink, D.C. and Raskin, P.M. (eds) (1996) *The Psychotherapy of Carl Rogers: Cases and Commentary*. New York: Guilford Press.

Feldmar, A. (1997) Contribution in B. Mullan (ed.) *R.D. Laing: Creative Destroyer*. London: Cassell.

Feltham, C. and Dryden, W. (1993) *Dictionary of Counselling*. London: Whurr.

Ferenczi, S. and Rank, O. (1925) *The Development of Psychoanalysis: Interrelations between Theory and Practice*. New York and Washington, D.C.: Nervous and Mental Disease Publishing Co.

Field, N. (1996) *Breakdown and Breakthrough*. London: Routledge.

Fizdale, R. (1958) Peer-group supervision, *Social Casework*, 39: 443–50.

Fleming, J. and Weiss, S.S. (1978) Assessment of progress in a training analysis, *International Review of Psycho-Analysis*, 5: 33–43.

Fliess, R. (1942) The metapsychology of the analyst, *Psychoanalytic Quarterly*, 11: 211–27.

Fordham, M. (1969) Countertransference and technique, in M. Fordham, R. Gordon, J. Hubback and K. Lambert (eds) (1974) *Technique in Jungian Analysis*. London: Heinemann.

Fordham, M. (1979) Analytical psychology and countertransference, in L. Epstein and A. Feiner (eds) *Counter-transference*. New York: Jason Aronson.

Fordham, M., Gordon, R., Hubback, J. and Lambert, K. (eds) (1974) *Technique in Jungian Analysis*, Vol. 2. The Library of Analytical Psychology. London: Heinemann.

Forsyth, D.R and Ivey, A.E. (1980) Microtraining: an approach to differential supervision, in A.K. Hess (ed.) *Psychotherapy Supervision: Theory, Research and Practice*. New York: Wiley.

Foulkes, S.H. and Anthony, E.J. (1965) *Group Psychotherapy: The Psychoanalytic Approach*, 2nd edn. London: Penguin.

Freud, S. (1910) The future prospects of psycho-analytic therapy, *Standard Edition*, Vol. 11. London: Hogarth Press.

Freud, S. (1912a) The dynamics of transference, *Standard Edition*, Vol. 12. London: Hogarth Press.

Freud, S. (1912b) Recommendations to physicians practicing psychoanalysis, *Standard Edition*, Vol. 12. London: Hogarth Press.

Freud, S. (1915) Observations on transference-love. (Further recommendations on the technique of psycho-analysis III), *Standard Edition*, Vol. 12. London: Hogarth Press.

Freud, S. (1916) Some character types met with in psychoanalytic work, *Standard Edition*, Vol. 14. London: Hogarth Press.

Freud, S. (1919) Lines of advance in psychoanalytic therapy, *Standard Edition*, Vol. 17. London: Hogarth Press.

Freud, S. (1921) *Group Psychology and the Analysis of the Ego*. Pelican Freud Library Vol. 12. London: Penguin.

Freud, S. (1923) Two encyclopaedia articles, *Standard Edition*, Vol. 18. London: Hogarth Press.

Freud, S. (1937) Analysis terminable and interminable, *International Journal of Psycho-Analysis*, 18: 373–405.

Freud, S. and Breuer, J. (1895) *Studies on Hysteria*. Pelican Freud Library Vol. 3. London: Penguin.

Friedenberg, E.Z. (1973) *Laing*. London: Fontana/Collins.

Friedman, M. (1976) Healing through meeting: a dialogic approach to psychotherapy and family therapy, in E. Smith (ed.) *Psychiatry and the Humanities*, Vol. 1. New Haven, CT: Yale University Press.

Friedman, M. (1996) Becoming aware: a dialogical approach to consciousness, *The Humanistic Psychologist*, 24: 203–20.

Fromm, E. (1956) *The Art of Loving*. New York: Harper & Row.

Fromm, E., Suzuki, D. and DiMartino, R. (1960) *Zen Buddhism and Psychoanalysis*. New York: Harper & Row.

Fruzzetti, A.E., Waltz, J.A. and Linehan, M.M. (1997) Supervision in dialectical behavior therapy, in C.E. Watkins (ed.) *Handbook of Psychotherapy Supervision*. New York: Wiley.

Fukuyama, M.B. and Sevig, T.D. (1999) *Integrating Spirituality into Multicultural Counseling*. Thousand Oaks, CA: Sage.

Gale, D. (1999) The limitations of boundaries, in C. Feltham (ed.) *Controversies in Psychotherapy and Counselling*. London: Sage.

Gaskill, H.S. (1980) The closing phase of the psychoanalytic treatment of adults and the goals of psychoanalysis, 'the myth of perfectibility', *International Journal of Psycho-Analysis*, 61: 11–22.

Gendlin, E.T. (1981) *Focusing*. New York: Bantam.

Gill, M.M. (1982) A method for studying the analysis of aspects of the patient's experience of the relationship in psychoanalysis and psychotherapy, *Journal of the American Psychoanalytic Association*, 30: 137–67.

Gilligan, C. (1982) *In a Different Voice: Psychological Theory and Women's Development*. Cambridge, MA: Harvard University Press.

Gitelson, M. (1952) The emotional position of the analyst in the psychoanalytic situation, *International Journal of Psycho-Analysis*, 35: 174–83.

Grant, J. and Crawley, J. (2002) *Transference and Projection*. Buckingham: Open University Press.

Greenberg, J. (1995) Self-disclosure: is it psychoanalytic?, *Contemporary Psychoanalysis*, 31: 193–205.

Groesbeck, C.J. (1975) The archetypal image of the wounded healer, *Journal of Analytical Psychology*, 20(2): 122–45.

Grof, C. and Grof, S. (1990) *The Stormy Search for the Self*. Los Angeles, CA: Tarcher.

Grof, S. (1988) *The Adventure of Self-discovery*. Albany, NY: State University of New York Press.

Grotstein, J.S. (1994) Projective identification and countertransference: a brief commentary on their relationship, *Contemporary Psychoanalysis*, 30: 578–92.

Guggenbühl-Craig, A. (1971) *Power in the Helping Professions*. New York: Spring.

Guntrip, H.J.S. (1968) *Schizoid Phenomena, Object Relations and the Self*. London: Hogarth Press.

Guntrip, H.J.S. (1975) My experience of analysis with Fairbairn and Winnicott, *International Review of Psycho-Analysis*, 2: 145–56.

Guntrip, H.J.S. (1996) My experience of analysis with Fairbairn and Winnicott, *International Journal of Psycho-Analysis*, 77: 739–54.

Hamburg, P. (1991) Interpretation and empathy: reading Lacan with Kohut, *International Journal of Psycho-Analysis*, 72: 347–61.

Hann-Kende, F. (1933) On the role of transference and countertransference in psychoanalysis, in G. Devereux (ed.) (1953) *Psychoanalysis and the Occult*. New York: International Universities Press.

Hart, T. (1997) Transcendental empathy in the therapeutic encounter, *The Humanistic Psychologist*, 25(3): 245–70.

Hart, T. (1998) Inspiration: exploring the experience and its meaning, *Journal of Humanistic Psychology*, 38(3): 7–35.

Hart, T. (1999) The refinement of empathy, *Journal of Humanistic Psychology*, 39(4): 111–25.

Hart, T. (2000) Deep empathy, in T. Hart, K. Puhakka and P. Nelson (eds) *Transpersonal Knowing: Exploring the Horizon of Consciousness*. Albany, NY: State University of New York Press.

Hattie, J.A., Sharpley, C.F. and Rogers, H.J. (1984) Comparative effectiveness of professional and paraprofessional helpers, *Psychological Bulletin*, 95: 534–41.

Haugh, S. and Merry, T. (eds) (2001) *Rogers' Therapeutic Conditions, Vol. 2: Empathy*. Ross-on-Wye: PCCS Books.

Hawkins, P. and Shohet, R. (2000) *Supervision in the Helping Professions*, 2nd edn. Buckingham: Open University Press.

Hazler, R. and Barwick, N. (2001) *The Therapeutic Environment*. Buckingham: Open University Press.

Heard, W.G. (1995) The unconscious functions of the I–It and I–Thou realms, *Humanistic Psychologist*, 23(2): 239–58.

Heidegger, M. (1962) *Being and Time* (trans. J. McQuarrie and E. Robinson). New York: Harper & Row.

Heidegger, M. (1993) The end of philosophy and the task of thinking, in D. Krell (ed.) *Martin Heidegger: Basic Writings*, 2nd edn. New York: HarperCollins.

Heimann, P. (1950) On counter-transference, *International Journal of Psycho-Analysis*, 31: 81–4.

Henderson, D. (1998) Solitude and solidarity: a philosophy of supervision, in P. Clarkson (ed.) *Supervision: Psychoanalytic and Jungian Perspectives*. London: Whurr.

Henderson, J.L. (1995) Assessing progress in supervision, in P. Kugler (ed.) *Jungian Perspectives on Clinical Supervision*. Einsiedeln: Daimon.

Henry, W.P., Strupp, H.H., Butler, S.F., Schacht, T.E. and Binder, J.L. (1993) Effects of training in time-limited dynamic psychotherapy: changes in therapist behavior, *Journal of Consulting and Clinical Psychology*, 61: 434–40.

Hess, A.K. (1980) Training models and the nature of psychotherapy supervision, in A.K. Hess (ed.) *Psychotherapy Supervision: Theory, Research and Practice*. New York: Wiley.

Hill, C.E. (1989) *Therapist Techniques and Client Outcomes: Eight Cases of Brief Psychotherapy*. Newbury Park, CA: Sage.

Hill, J. (1993) Am I a Kleinian? Is anyone?, *British Journal of Psychotherapy*, 9(4): 463–75.

Hillman, J. (1973/1990) *Suicide and the Soul*. Dallas, TX: Spring.

Hillman, J. (1975) *Re-visioning Psychology*. New York: Harper Colophon.

Hillman, J. (1979) Puer's wound and Ulysses's scar, in *Puer Papers*. Dallas, TX: Spring.

Hillman, J. (1996) *The Soul's Code*. London: Bantam Books.

Hinshelwood, R.D. (1989) *A Dictionary of Kleinian Thought*. London: Free Association Press.

Hoffer, A. (1985) Toward a definition of psychoanalytic neutrality, *Journal of the American Psychoanalytic Association*, 33: 771–95.

Hoffer, W. (1956) Transference and transference neurosis, *International Journal of Psycho-Analysis*, 37: 377–9.

Hoffman, I.Z. (1992) Expressive participation and psychoanalytic discipline, *Contemporary Psychoanalysis*, 28: 1–15.

Hoffman, I.Z. (1994) Dialectical thinking and therapeutic action in the psychoanalytic process, *Psychoanalytic Quarterly*, 63: 187–218.

Hoffman, M.L. (1990) Empathy and justice motivation, *Motivation and Emotion*, 14(2): 151–72.

Holloway, E. (1995) *Clinical Supervision: A Systems Approach*. Thousand Oaks, CA: Sage.

House, R. and Totton, N. (eds) (1997) *Implausible Professions: Arguments for Pluralism and Autonomy in Psychotherapy and Counselling*. Ross-on-Wye: PCCS Books.

Houston, G. (1995) *Supervision and Counselling* (revised edition). London: Rochester Foundation.

Husserl, E. ([1929]1967) *The Paris Lectures*. The Hague: Martinus Nijhoff.

Hycner, R. (1993) *Between Person and Person: Toward a Dialogical Psychotherapy*. Highland, NY: Gestalt Journal Press.

Inskipp, F. (2000) Generic skills, in C. Feltham and I. Horton (eds) *Handbook of Counselling and Psychotherapy*. London: Sage.

Ivey, A.E., Ivey, M.B. and Simek-Downing, L. (1987) *Counseling and Psychotherapy: Integrating Skills, Theory and Practice*, 2nd edn. Englewood Cliffs, NJ: Prentice-Hall.

Jacobs, M. (1996) Parallel process – confirmation and critique, *Journal of Psychodynamic Counselling*, 2(1): 55–66.

Jacobs, M. (2000a) *Illusion: A Psychodynamic Interpretation of Thinking and Belief*. London: Whurr.

Jacobs, M. (2000b) *Swift to Hear: Facilitating Skills in Listening and Responding*. London: SPCK.

Jacobs, M. (2001) Reflections (psychodynamic psychotherapy), in E. Spinelli and S. Marshall (eds) *Embodied Theories*. London: Continuum.

Jacobs, T.J. (1999) Countertransference past and present: a review of the concept, *International Journal of Psycho-Analysis*, 80: 575–94.

James, V. (1996) Dreaming. Unpublished dissertation, The Minster Centre; London.

Jones, E. (1955) *Sigmund Freud: Life and Work*, Vol. 2. London: Hogarth Press.

Jourard, S.M. (1968) *Disclosing Man to Himself*. Princeton, NJ: Van Nostrand.

Jourard, S.M. (1971) *The Transparent Self*, 2nd edn. New York: Van Nostrand Reinhold.

Jukes, A. (1993) *Why Men Hate Women*. London: Free Association Books.

Jung, C.G. (1966) The practice of psychotherapy, in *Collected Works*, Vol. 16, 2nd edn. London: Routledge & Kegan Paul.

Jung, C.G. (1968) *Collected Works*, Vol. 7. London: Routledge.

Kennedy, E. and Charles, C. (1989) *On Becoming a Counsellor*, 2nd edn. Dublin: Gill & Macmillan.

Kernberg, O. (1975) *Borderline Conditions and Pathological Narcissism*. New York: Jason Aronson.

Kernberg, O.F. (1986) Institutional problems of psychoanalytic education, *Journal of American Psychoanalytic Association*, 34: 799–834.

Kernberg, O.F. (1996) Thirty methods to destroy the creativity of psycho-analytic candidates, *International Journal of Psycho-Analysis*, 77: 1031–40.

Khan, M.M.R. (1974) *The Privacy of the Self*. New York: International Universities Press.

King, L. (ed.) (1999) *Committed Uncertainty in Psychotherapy: Essays in Honour of Peter Lomas*. London: Whurr.

King, M. (2000) Examining therapists' rationale for self-disclosure, Research dissertation, Surrey University.

King-Spooner, S. and Newnes, C. (2001) *Spirituality and Psychotherapy*. Ross-on-Wye: PCCS Books.

Kohlberg, L. (1981) *The Philosophy of Moral Development*. San Francisco, CA: Harper & Row.

Kohn, A. (1990) *The Brighter Side of Human Existence: Altruism and Empathy in Everyday Life*. New York: Basic Books.

Kohut, H. (1980a) Reflections, in A. Goldberg (ed.) *Advances in Self Psychology*. New York: International Universities Press.

Kohut, H. (1980b) Two letters, in A. Goldberg (ed.) *Advances in Self Psychology*. New York: International Universities Press.

Kohut, H. (1984) *How Does Analysis Cure?* Chicago, IL: University of Chicago Press.

Kovacs, V. (1936) Training- and control-analysis, *International Journal of Psycho-Analysis*, 17: 346–54.

Kramer, C.H. (2000) Revealing our selves, in M. Baldwin (ed.) *The Use of Self in Therapy*, 2nd edn. Binghamton: Haworth Press.

Kratochwill, T.R., Lepage, K.M. and McGivern, J. (1997) Child and adolescent psychotherapy supervision, in C.E. Watkins (ed.) *Handbook of Psychotherapy Supervision*. New York: Wiley.

Laing, R.D. (1962) *The Self and Others*. London: Tavistock.

Laing, R.D. (1982) *The Voice of Experience*. London: Penguin.

Lake, F. (1966) *Clinical Theology*. London: Darton, Longman & Todd.

Lake, F. (1980) *Constricted Confusion*. Oxford: Clinical Theology Association.

Lander, N.R. and Nahon, D. (2000) Personhood of the therapist in couples therapy: an integrity therapy perspective, in B.J. Brothers (ed.) *The Personhood of the Therapist*. Binghamton, NY: Haworth Press.

Langs, R.J. (1980) Supervision and the bipersonal field, in A.K. Hess (ed.) *Psychotherapy Supervision: Theory, Research and Practice*. New York: Wiley.

Langs, R. (1982) *Psychotherapy: A Basic Text*. New York: Jason Aronson.

Lapworth, P. (1995) Transactional analysis, in M. Jacobs (ed.) *Charlie: An Unwanted Child?* Buckingham: Open University Press.

Larson, V.A. (1987) An exploration of psychotherapeutic resonance, *Psychotherapy*, 24(3): 321–4.

Lazarus, A.A. (1989) *The Practice of Multimodal Therapy*. Baltimore, MD: Johns Hopkins University Press.

Lewin, K. (1963) *Field Theory in Social Science: Selected Theoretical Papers*. London: Tavistock.

Lewis, C.S. (1960) *The Four Loves*. New York: Harcourt Brace.

Lidmila, A. (1997) Shame, knowledge and modes of enquiry in supervision, in G. Shipton (ed.) *Supervision of Psychotherapy and Counselling*. Buckingham: Open University Press.

Linehan, M.M. (1980) Supervision of behaviour therapy, in A.K. Hess (ed.) *Psychotherapy Supervision: Theory, Research and Practice*. New York: Wiley.

Liss, J. (1996) The identification approach, *Energy and Character*, 27: 45–60.

Little, M.I. (1951) Countertransference and the patient's response to it, *International Journal of Psycho-Analysis*, 32: 32–40.

Little, M.I. (1990) *Psychotic Anxieties and Containment: A Personal Record of an Analysis with Winnicott*. New York: Jason Aronson.

Loevinger, J. (1976) *Ego Development*. San Francisco, CA: Jossey-Bass.

Lomas, P. (1973) *True and False Experience*. London: Allen Lane.

Lomas, P. (1981) *The Case for a Personal Psychotherapy*. Oxford: Oxford University Press.

Lomas, P. (1994) *Cultivating Intuition: An Introduction to Psychotherapy*. London: Penguin.

Lomas, P. (1999) *Doing Good?: Psychotherapy out of its Depth*. Oxford: Oxford University Press.

Maclagan, D. (1997) Fantasy, play and the image in supervision, in G. Shipton (ed.) *Supervision of Psychotherapy and Counselling*. Buckingham: Open University Press.

Maguire, K. (2001) Working with survivors of torture and extreme experiences, in S. King-Spooner and C. Newnes (eds) *Spirituality and Psychotherapy*. Ross-on-Wye: PCCS Books.

Mahrer, A.R. (1983) *Experiential Psychotherapy*. New York: Brunner/Mazel.

Mahrer, A.R. (1989) *How to do Experiential Psychotherapy: A Manual for Practitioners*. Ottawa: University of Ottawa Press.

Mahrer, A.R. (1996) *The Complete Guide to Experiential Psychotherapy*. New York: Wiley.

Mahrer, A.R. (1998) Embarrassing problems for the field of psychotherapy, *Psychotherapy Section Newsletter*, 23: 19–29.

Mahrer, A.R., Boulet, D.B. and Fairweather, D.R. (1994) Beyond empathy: advances in the clinical theory and methods of empathy, *Clinical Psychology Review*, 14: 183–98.

Malan, D.H. (1979) *Individual Psychotherapy and the Science of Psychodynamics*. London: Butterworth.

Margison, F. (1995) Psychoanalytic psychotherapy, in M. Jacobs (ed.) *Charlie: An Unwanted Child?* Buckingham: Open University Press.

Maslow, A.H. (1968) *Toward a Psychology of Being*, 2nd edn. New York: Van Nostrand.

Maslow, A.H. (1987) *Motivation and Personality*, 3rd edn. New York: Harper & Row.

Masson, J.M. (ed.) (1985) *The Complete Letters of Sigmund Freud to Wilhelm Fliess 1887–1904*. Cambridge, MA: Belknap Press.

Maupin, E.W. (1965) Zen Buddhism: a psychological review, *Journal of Counselling Psychology*, 29: 139–45.

May, R. (1980) *Psychology and the Human Dilemma.* New York: W.W. Norton.

May, R. (1983) *The Discovery of Being.* New York: W.W. Norton.

McGuire, W. (1974) *The Freud/Jung Letters.* London: Hogarth Press/Routledge & Kegan Paul.

Mearns, D. (1994) *Developing Person-Centred Counselling.* London: Sage.

Mearns, D. (1996) Working at relational depth with clients in person-centred therapy, *Counselling,* 7(4): 306–11.

Mearns, D. (1997) *Person-Centred Counselling Training.* London: Sage.

Mearns, D. and Thorne, B. (1988) *Person-Centred Counselling in Action.* London: Sage.

Mearns, D. and Thorne, B. (2000) *Person-Centred Therapy Today: New Frontiers for Theory and Practice.* London: Sage.

Menzies, I.E.P. (1960) A case study in the functioning of a social system as a defence against anxiety, *International Journal of Therapeutic Communities,* 6: 37–44.

Millar, A. (1995) Adlerian therapy, in M. Walker (ed.) *Morag: Myself or Mother-hen?* Buckingham: Open University Press.

Miller, G.D. and Baldwin, D.C. (2000) Implications of the wounded-healer paradigm for the use of self in therapy, in M. Baldwin (ed.) *The Use of Self in Therapy,* 2nd edn. Binghamton, NY: Haworth Press.

Milner, M. (1987) *The Suppressed Madness of Sane Men.* London: Routledge.

Money-Kyrle, R. (1956) Normal counter-transference and some of its deviations, in *The Collected Works of Roger Money-Kyrle.* Strath Tay: Clunie Press.

Moreno, Z.T., Blomkvist, L.D. and Rutzel, T. (2000) *Psychodrama, Surplus Reality and the Art of Healing.* London: Routledge.

Mowbray, R. (1995) *The Case Against Psychotherapy Registration: A Conservation Issue for the Human Potential Movement.* London: Transmarginal Press.

Mullan, B. (1995) *Mad to be Normal: Conversations with R.D. Laing.* London: Free Association Books.

Myss, C. (1996) *Anatomy of Spirit: The Seven Stages of Power and Healing.* New York: Harmony Books.

Nelson, J.E. (1994) *Healing the Split: Integrating Spirit into Our Understanding of the Mentally Ill.* Albany, NY: State University of New York Press.

Nuttall, J. (2000) Modes of therapeutic relationship in Kleinian psychotherapy, *British Journal of Psychotherapy,* 17(1): 17–36.

Obholzer, K. (1980) *The Wolf-Man.* London: Routledge & Kegan Paul.

Orbach, S. (1995) Countertransference and the false body, *Winnicott Studies,* 10: 3–13.

Ormrod, J. (1995) Cognitive behaviour therapy, in M. Walker (ed.) *Peta: A Feminist's Problem with Men.* Buckingham: Open University Press.

Padesky, C.A. (1996) Developing cognitive therapist competency: teaching and supervision models, in P.M. Salkovskis (ed.) *Frontiers of Cognitive Therapy.* New York: Guilford Press.

Page, S. (1999) *The Shadow and the Counsellor.* London: Routledge.

Page, S. and Wosket, V. (1994) *Supervising the Counsellor: A Cyclical Model.* London: Routledge.

Phillips, E.L. (1951) Attitudes toward self and others: a brief questionnaire report, *Journal of Consulting Psychology*, 15: 79–81.

Piaget, J. (1950) *The Psychology of Intelligence*. London: Routledge & Kegan Paul.

Poland, W.S. (1984) On the analyst's neutrality, *Journal of the American Psychoanalytic Association*, 32: 283–99.

Polster, E. and Polster, M. (1973) *Gestalt Therapy Integrated*. New York: Vintage Books.

Puhakka, K. (2000) An invitation to authentic knowing, in T. Hart, P.L. Nelson and K. Puhakka (eds) *Transpersonal Knowing: Exploring the Horizon of Consciousness*. Albany, NY: State University of New York Press.

Rabin, B. and Walker, R. (undated) *A Contemplative Approach to Clinical Supervision*. Boulder, CO: Naropa Institute.

Racker, H. (1957) The meanings and uses of countertransference, *Psychoanalytic Quarterly*, 26: 303–57.

Racker, H. (1968) *Transference and Countertransference*. London: Hogarth Press.

Rangell, L. (1954) Similarities and differences between psychoanalysis and dynamic psychotherapy, *Journal of the American Psychoanalytic Association*, 2: 734–44.

Reich, A. (1951) On counter-transference, *International Journal of Psycho-Analysis*, 32: 25–31.

Renik, O. (1995) The ideal of the anonymous analyst and the problem of self-disclosure, *Psychoanalytic Quarterly*, 64: 466–95.

Rice, L.N. (1980) A client-centred approach to the supervision of psychotherapy, in A.K. Hess (ed.) *Psychotherapy Supervision: Theory, Research and Practice*. New York: Wiley.

Ricketts, T. and Donohoe, G. (2000) Supervision in cognitive behavioural psychotherapy, in B. Lawton and C. Feltham (eds) *Taking Supervision Forward*. London: Sage.

Rioch, M.J., Coulter, W.R. and Weinberger, D.M. (1976) *Dialogues for Therapists*. San Francisco, CA: Jossey-Bass.

Rogers, C.R. (1957) The necessary and sufficient conditions of therapeutic personality change, *Journal of Consulting Psychology*, 21(2): 99.

Rogers, C.R. (1980) *A Way of Being*. Boston, MA: Houghton Mifflin.

Rogers, C.R. (1986) A client-centered, person-centered approach to therapy, in L. Kutash and A. Wolf (eds) *A Psychotherapist's Casebook: Therapy and Technique in Practice*. San Francisco, CA: Jossey-Bass.

Ross, M. (2000) Body talk: somatic countertransference, *Journal of Psychodynamic Counselling*, 6(4): 51–67.

Rowan, J. (1986) Holistic listening, *Journal of Humanistic Psychology*, 26(1): 83–102.

Rowan, J. (1993) *The Transpersonal: Psychotherapy and Counselling*. London: Routledge.

Rowan, J. (1998a) *The Reality Game: A Guide to Humanistic Counselling and Psychotherapy*, 2nd edn. London: Routledge.

Rowan, J. (1998b) Linking: its place in therapy, *International Journal of Psychotherapy*, 3(3): 245–54.

Rowan, J. (2000) Back to basics: two kinds of therapy, *Counselling*, 21(2): 76–8.

Rowan, J. (2001a) Supervision and the psychospiritual levels of development, *Transpersonal Psychology Review*, 5(2): 12–21.

Rowan, J. (2001b) *Ordinary Ecstasy: The Dialectics of Humanistic Psychology*, 3rd edn. London: Brunner/Routledge.

Russell, R. (1981) *Report on Effective Psychotherapy: Legislative Testimony*. New York: RR Latin Associates.

Russell, R. (1993) *Report on Effective Psychotherapy: Legislative Testimony*. New York: Hilgarth Press (endorsed by the American Psychological Association).

Rycroft, C. (ed.) (1968) *Psychoanalysis Observed*. London: Penguin.

Rycroft, C. (1985) *Psychoanalysis and Beyond*. London: Chatto & Windus.

Ryle, A. (1995) Cognitive-analytic therapy, in M. Jacobs (ed.) *Charlie: An Unwanted Child?* Buckingham: Open University Press.

Samuels, A. (1985) *Jung and the Post-Jungians*. London: Routledge & Kegan Paul.

Samuels, A. (1989) *The Plural Psyche*. London: Routledge.

Samuels, A. (1993) *The Political Psyche*. London: Routledge.

Samuels, A. (1997) Countertransference, the imaginal world and the politics of the sublime, in P. Clarkson (ed.) *On the Sublime: In Psychoanalysis, Archetypal Psychology and Psychotherapy*. London: Whurr.

Sandler, A.-M. (1982) The selection and function of the training analyst in Europe, *International Review of Psycho-Analysis*, 9: 386–98.

Sandler, J., Dare, C. and Holder, A. (1973) *The Patient and the Analyst*. London: George Allen & Unwin.

Sapriel, L. (1998) Can Gestalt therapy, self-psychology and intersubjectivity theory be integrated?, *British Gestalt Journal*, 7(1): 33–44.

Sartre, J.-P. (1948) *Existentialism and Humanism*. London: Methuen.

Satir, V. (1987) quoted in Satir, V. (2000) The personhood of the therapist: effect on systems, in B.J. Brothers (ed.) *The Personhood of the Therapist*. New York: Haworth Press.

Schachter, J. (1994) Abstinence and neutrality: development and diverse views, *International Journal of Psycho-Analysis*, 75: 709–20.

Schwartz-Salant, N. (1984), in N. Schwartz-Salant and M. Stein (eds) *Transference, Counter-transference*. Wilmette: Chiron.

Schwartz-Salant, N. (1991), in N. Schwartz-Salant and M. Stein (eds) *Liminality and Transitional Phenomena*. Wilmette: Chiron.

Searles, H.F. (1955) The informational value of the supervisor's emotional experiences, in H.F. Searles (1965) *Collected Papers on Schizophrenia and Related Subjects*. London: Hogarth Press/Karnac Press.

Searles, H.F. (1959) Oedipal love in the counter-transference, in H.F. Searles (1965) *Collected Papers on Schizophrenia and Related Subjects*. London: Hogarth Press/Karnac Press.

Searles, H.F. (1962) Problems of psycho-analytic supervision, in H.F. Searles (1965) *Collected Papers on Schizophrenia and Related Subjects*. London: Hogarth Press/Karnac Press.

Searles, H.F. (1965) *Collected Papers on Schizophrenia and Related Subjects.* London: Hogarth Press/Karnac Press.

Searles, H.F. (1972) The patient as therapist to his analyst, in H.F. Searles (1979) *Countertransference and Related Subjects.* New York: International Universities Press.

Searles, H.F. (1979) *Countertransference and Related Subjects.* New York: International Universities Press.

Searles, H.F. with Bisco, J.M., Coutu, G. and Scibetta, R.C. (1973) Violence in schizophrenia, in H.F. Searles (1979) *Countertransference and Related Subjects.* New York: International Universities Press.

Sedgwick, D. (1993) *Jung and Searles: A Comparative Analysis.* London: Routledge.

Segal, H. (1964) *Introduction to the Work of Melanie Klein.* New York: Basic Books.

Seguin, C.A. (1965) *Love and Psychotherapy.* New York: Libra.

Seiser, L. and Wastell, C. (2002) *Interventions and Techniques.* Buckingham: Open University Press.

Shadley, M.L. (2000) Are all therapists alike? Revisiting research about the use of self in therapy, in M. Baldwin (ed.) *The Use of Self in Therapy*, 2nd edn. New York: Haworth Press.

Shapiro, T.C. (1984) On neutrality, *Journal of the American Psychoanalytic Association*, 32: 269–82.

Sheldrake, R. (1988) *The Presence of the Past: Morphic Resonance and the Habits of Nature.* New York: Vintage.

Sherman, D. (1945) An analysis of the dynamic relationships between counsellor techniques and outcomes in larger units of the interview situation, unpublished doctoral dissertation, Ohio State University.

Simanowitz, V. and Pearce, P. (forthcoming) *Personality Development.* Buckingham: Open University Press.

Singer, E. (1977) The fiction of analytic anonymity, in K.A. Frank (ed.) *The Human Dimension in Psychoanalysis.* New York: Grune & Stratton.

Slack, S. (1985) Reflections on a workshop with Carl Rogers, *Journal of Humanistic Psychology*, 28: 35–42.

Smith, E.W.L., Clance, P.R. and Imes, S. (1998) *Touch in Psychotherapy: Theory, Research and Practice.* New York: Guilford Press.

Smith, N.L. and Smith, L.L. (1996) Field theory in science: its role as a necessary and sufficient condition in psychology, *Psychological Record*, 46: 3–19.

Snyder, M. (2000) The radical leap of true empathy: a case example, in B.J. Brothers (ed.) *The Personhood of the Therapist.* Binghamton, NY: Haworth Press.

Spinelli, E. (2001) *The Mirror and the Hammer: Challenges to Therapeutic Orthodoxy.* London: Continuum.

Spinelli, E. and Marshall, S. (eds) (2001) *Embodied Theories.* London: Continuum.

Sprinkle, L. (1985) Psychological resonance: a holographic model of counselling, *Journal of Counselling and Development*, 64: 206–8.

Sterling, M.M. and Bugental, J.F.T. (1993) The meld experience in psychotherapy supervision, *Journal of Humanistic Psychology*, 33(2): 38–48.

Stolorow, R.D. and Atwood, G. (1992) *Contexts of Being: The Intersubjective Foundations of Psychological Life*. Hillsdale, NJ: Analytic Press.

Sullivan, B.S. (1989) *Psychotherapy Grounded in the Feminine Principle*. Wilmette: Chiron.

Syme, G. and Elton Wilson, J. (forthcoming) *Aims and Outcomes*. Buckingham: Open University Press.

Symington, J. and Symington, N. (1996) *The Clinical Thinking of Wilfred Bion*. London: Routledge.

Tansey, M.J. and Burke, W.F. (1989) *Understanding Countertransference: From Projective Identification to Empathy*. Hillsdale, NJ: Analytic Press.

Thich Nhat Hanh (1995) *The Heart of Understanding: Commentaries on the Prajnaparamita Heart Sutra*. Berkeley, CA: Parallax Press.

Thorne, B.J. (1987) Beyond the core conditions, in W. Dryden (ed.) *Key Cases in Psychotherapy*. London: Croom Helm.

Tolpin, P. (1988) Optimal affective engagement: the analyst's role in therapy, in A. Goldberg (ed.) *Progress in Self Psychology*, Vol. 4. Hillsdale, NJ: Analytic Press.

Trop, J.L. and Stolorow, R.D. (1997) Therapeutic empathy: an intersubjective perspective, in A.C. Bohart and L.S. Greenberg (eds) *Empathy Reconsidered: New Directions in Psychotherapy*. Washington, DC: American Psychological Association.

Trower, P., Casey, A. and Dryden, W. (1988) *Cognitive Behavioural Counselling in Action*. London: Sage.

Tyson, R.L. (1986) Countertransference: evolution in theory and practice, *Journal of the American Psychoanalytic Association*, 34: 251–74.

van Deurzen-Smith, E. (1988) *Existential Counselling in Practice*. London: Sage.

Wade, J. (1996) *Changes of Mind: A Holonomic Theory of the Evolution of Consciousness*. Albany, NY: State University of New York Press.

Waelder, R. (1960) *Basic Theory of Psychoanalysis*. New York: International Universities Press.

Wallerstein, R.S. (1978) Perspectives on psychoanalytic training around the world, *International Journal of Psycho-Analysis*, 59: 477–503.

Wallerstein, R.S. (1988) One psychoanalysis or many?, *International Journal of Psycho-Analysis*, 69: 5–21.

Wallerstein, R.S. (1993) Between chaos and petrification: a summary of the fifth IPA Conference of Training Analysts, *International Journal of Psycho-Analysis*, 74: 165–78.

Wallis, K. and Poulton, J.L. (2001) *Internalization*. Buckingham: Open University Press.

Watkins, C.E., Jr. (1989) Countertransference: its impact on the counselling situation, in W. Dryden (ed.) *Key Issues in Counselling in Action*. London: Sage.

Watkins, J. (1978) *The Therapeutic Self*. New York: Human Sciences Press.

Watson, K.W. (1973) Differential supervision, *Social Work*, 18: 80–8.

Wellings, N. and McCormick, E.W. (2000) *Transpersonal Psychotherapy: Theory and Practice*. London: Continuum.

Wessler, R.L. and Ellis, A. (1980) Supervision in rational-emotive therapy, in A.K. Hess (ed.) *Psychotherapy Supervision: Theory, Research and Practice*. New York: Wiley.

West, W. (2000) *Psychotherapy and Spirituality*. London: Sage.

Wheeler, G. (1998) Towards a Gestalt developmental model, *British Gestalt Journal*, 7(2): 115–25.

Wheelwright, J.B. (1982) Termination, in M. Stein (ed.) *Jungian Analysis*. Boston, MA: Shambhala.

Wheway, J. (1997) Dialogue and intersubjectivity in the therapeutic relationship, *British Gestalt Journal*, 6(1): 16–28.

Whitmore, D. (1999) *Supervision from a Transpersonal Context* (unpublished document). London: Psychosynthesis and Education Trust.

Wilber, K. (1980a) *The Atman Project*. Wheaton: Quest.

Wilber, K. (1980b) The pre/trans fallacy, *ReVision*, 3: 2.

Wilber, K. (1981) *No Boundary*. London: Routledge.

Wilber, K. (1983) *A Sociable God*. New York: McGraw-Hill.

Wilber, K. (1995) *Sex, Ecology, Spirituality*. Boston, MA: Shambhala.

Wilber, K. (2000) *Integral Psychology*. Boston, MA: Shambhala.

Wilber, K., Engler, J. and Brown, D.P. (1986) *Transformations of Consciousness*. Boston, MA: Shambhala.

Winnicott, D.W. (1947) Hate in the countertransference, in D.W. Winnicott (1975) *Through Paediatrics to Psychoanalysis: Collected Papers*. London: Hogarth Press.

Winnicott, D.W. (1965) *The Maturational Processes and the Facilitating Environment*. London: Karnac Books.

Winnicott, D.W. (1971) *Playing and Reality*. London: Routledge.

Winnicott, D.W. (1975) *Through Paediatrics to Psychoanalysis: Collected Papers*. London: Karnac Books.

Winnicott, D.W. (1988) *Human Nature*. London: Free Association Books.

Wolf, E.S. (1988) *Treating the Self: Elements of Clinical Self Psychology*. New York: Guilford Press.

Yalom, I. (1989) *Love's Executioner*. London: Bloomsbury.

Yalom, I. and Elkin, G. (1974) *Every Day Gets a Little Closer: A Twice Told Therapy*. New York: Basic Books.

Yontef, G. (1993) *Awareness, Dialogue and Process: Essays on Gestalt Therapy*. Highland, NY: Gestalt Journal Press.

Yontef, G. (1997) Supervision from a Gestalt therapy perspective, in C.E. Watkins (ed.) *Handbook of Psychotherapy Supervision*. New York: Wiley.

Young-Eisendrath, P. and Miller, M.E. (2000) *The Psychology of Mature Spirituality: Integrity, Wisdom, Transcendence*. London: Routledge.

Zelen, S.L. (1954) Acceptance and acceptability, *Journal of Consulting Psychology*, 18: 316.

Zinker, J. (1978) *Creative Process in Gestalt Therapy*. New York: Vintage Books.

Index